# Rainbow
# Reiki

W9-CCT-799

Walter Lübeck

# Rainbow
# Reiki

Expanding the Reiki System
with Powerful Spiritual Abilities

LOTUS LIGHT
SHANGRI-LA

Reiki is an effective system for healing and stimulating mental, emotional, and spiritual growth. However, Reiki does not make the visit to a doctor, naturopath, or psychotherapist superfluous when there is a suspicion of a serious health disorder. Naturopathy (which also includes Reiki) would like to supplement orthodox medicine wherever the latter cannot heal people and animals, but it does not want to consider it unnecessary in any respect.

The information and exercises introduced in my book have been carefully researched and passed on to the best of my knowledge and conscience. Despite this fact, the author and the publisher do not assume any type of liability for damages of any type which occur through the direct or indirect application or utilization of the statements in this book.

*A further note:* The illustrations in this book show nude people in order to graphically demonstrate the hand positions of Reiki and better convey the atmosphere of closeness, freedom, and love which Reiki radiates. But this does not mean that Reiki must be practiced in the nude. Participants in the Reiki training seminars are also fully dressed.

When I talk about the Master, Grand Master, and students, the feminine form of these words is fundamentally included as well. When the word "he" is used in place of the more awkward "he or she," it is not meant to be discriminatory in any way.

The terms Rainbow Reiki™, Rainbow Reiki Essence™, and Rainbow Reiki Mandala™ can be freely used by private individuals. However, these are protected trademarks and not to be applied for commercial purposes with the express permission of the author.

1st English edition 1997
© Lotus Light Publications, P. O. Box 325, Twin Lakes, WI 53181
The Shangri-La Series is published in cooperation with Schneelöwe Verlagsberatung, Federal Republic of Germany
©1994 reserved by Windpferd Verlagsgesellschaft mbH, Aitrang
All rights reserved
Translated by Christine M. Grimm
Cover design by Wolfgang Jünemann
Illustrations by Roland Tietsch
ISBN 0-914955-28-4
Library of Congress Catalog Number 97-71446

Printed in the USA

# Table of Contents

*Introduction*                                                                 9

CHAPTER ONE
*Fundamentals of Rainbow Reiki*                                                13
The Usui System of Reiki as the Basis for Rainbow Reiki                        13
Preconditions for the Practice
of Rainbow Reiki in the First Degree                                          14
Preconditions for the Practice
of Rainbow Reiki in the Second Degree                                         15
According to Which Laws Does
Rainbow Reiki Function?                                                        15
What is Healing?                                                               18
The Three Steps of Holistic Healing                                           18
The Three Components of Genuine Spiritual Development                          19
Rainbow Reiki Principles for Energy Work
and Life Improvement                                                          21
Responsibility—An Important Topic
in Relation to Rainbow Reiki                                                  23
The Light Vow Ritual                                                          24

CHAPTER TWO
*Aura and Chakra Work with Rainbow Reiki*                                      27
How You Can Deal with Healing Reactions...                                    27
How You as a Practitioner Can Deal with Imbalances
That You Take On from Your Clients                                            28

CHAPTER THREE
*Rainbow Reiki Mandalas—Healing Patterns*
*That Help Bring Light and Love to the Earth*                                  39
The Story of the Rainbow Reiki Mandala Method's Origin                        39
Hey Loa, Key Loa, Manaho Lo—An Old Healing Song
and Its Various Effects                                                       40
Rainbow Reiki Plant Mandalas                                                  41
Rainbow Reiki Crystal Mandalas                                                43
The Four Main Chakra Healing Mandalas                                         47
Examples for Practical Applications of the
Rainbow Reiki Mandalas                                                        53

CHAPTER FOUR
*Rainbow Reiki and Work with*
*Friends from the Subtle Dimensions*                                    55
Subtle Beings Aren't "Substitute Gods"                                  57
Theoretical Foundations for Contacts
and Work with Subtle Beings                                            57
The Iceberg Principle: Your Everyday Life Happens
at the Focus of Your Consciousness Work                                58
Subtle Helper Forces—The Invisible Friends                             59
Human Beings Also Have Subtle Portions with
Immense Hidden Powers                                                  60
Reiki as an Offering                                                   66
Addressing Subtle Beings in an Appropriate Manner                      67
Contact Training with Angels, Medicine Animals,
and Other Exotic Friends                                               67
Reiki and Your Higher Self                                             71
Hidden Knowledge in Plants and Minerals                                79
Some Examples for Practical Uses
of Work with Subtle Beings                                             79

CHAPTER FIVE
*Rainbow Reiki and Energy Work with Power Places*                      83
General Information on Power Places                                     83
The Differing Qualities of the Power Places                            84
Various Categories of Power Places                                     86
How You Can Meaningfully Work with
Power Places                                                          93
Basic Exercises for Power Place Work                                   93
Recognizing and Learning to Use the Various
Work Areas of a Power Place                                            97
Gifts You Can Receive from a Power Place                              103
Cross-Linking Power Places with Each Other                            103
How You Can Set Up a Power Place                                      105
Why New Power Places Should Be Established                            107

CHAPTER SIX
*Reiki Essences—A New Method for Discovering*
*the Healing Powers of Nature for Yourself*                           109
The History of Reiki Essences                                         109
The Theoretical Background of Reiki Essences                          110
Who Can Make Reiki Essences?                                          111
Preparing to Make Reiki Essences
with Reiki and Meditation                                             112
Making Reiki Essences in General                                      114
Reiki Essence Dosage                                                  116

Examples of Preparation and Effect
of Various Reiki Essences                                116
Examples of Proven Transformation Essences               118
How Can Reiki Essences Be Used Everywhere
and What Should Be Observed in the Process?              126
An Application of the Reiki Essence Method
for Advanced Students                                    126

CHAPTER SEVEN
*Reiki Essences in Practical Application*                 129
What Happens When Reiki Essences Are Used?               129
What are Healing Reactions?                              129
Social Impact of Taking Reiki Essences                  130
When You Should See a Doctor?                           131
Interaction of Reiki Essences
with Other Medications                                  131
Reiki Essences and Regulations                          132
One Reservation on My Part...                           132
Certification Training at the Reiki-Do Institute        133
Training for Non-Professionals in the Reiki Essence
Method                                                  133

APPENDIX ONE
*A Brief Explanation of the Four Aura Fields
and Seven Major Chakras*                                 135

APPENDIX TWO
*Experiences with Reiki Essences*
*(by Anne Witt, Healing Practitioner and Reiki Master)*  139
General Observations on the Reiki Essences              148

APPENDIX THREE
*Reiki, Shamanism, and Working with the
Healing Powers of Nature*
*(By Greta-Bahya Hessel-Lübeck)*                         149
What Is Shamanism?                                      149
What Shamanism Isn't                                   150
My Path with the Powers                                 150
The "Medicine Cards" in Personal Counseling
and Shamanistic Work                                    151

APPENDIX FOUR
*Pendulum Tables*                                        153

APPENDIX FIVE
*Commented Bibliography*                                 171

# Introduction

*Progress is the realization of utopias.*
(Oscar Wilde)

It's now been more than seven years since Reiki, or more precisely: the Usui System of Natural Healing, entered my life. Much has happened since then. Sometimes I have the feeling that I have lived a hundred years in this relatively short period of time when I let the many intense experiences pass through my mind. Yet, often when I become acquainted with a further possibility for applying this unique system of energy work (because I can't be discouraged from the thought that a certain thing can also somehow be accomplished with Reiki), it seems to me that I'm just getting to know it for the first time. So many new things occur with infallible regularity that I'm astonished over and over again. The intensive contact with this force on a regular basis in thousands of initiations, research, and treatments permits me to more strongly feel the highs—and the lows—of my life. Reiki gives me the strength to do important things and guides me, when I let it, on the right path to the experiences and perceptions that are important for me. As a result, this wonderful "universal" life energy has become a matter of course for me. This is true to such an extent that I often, even when I sleep, am involved with the Reiki symbols and mantras or lay my hands on my body and treat myself—as my wife tells me with a laugh in the morning.

On the other hand, I feel that the further my knowledge in relation to Reiki and energy work develops in general, the less I basically know. Then I realize how many fantastic possibilities are waiting to be explored and applied. There are still so many unsolved mysteries, and so I don't even want to stop exploring Rainbow Reiki. However, solely the fact *that* a certain Rainbow Reiki technique works isn't enough for me on its own. Since I like to take responsibility for what I do, it's important to me to comprehend *how* something functions, exactly what I'm doing, and why it produces certain effects, and under which circumstances something doesn't work. I pass on the results of this excursion through the world of Reiki to my students in the various advanced courses on the First, Second, and Third Degrees and am happy when they experience something wonderful with them. Many responses from this circle of enthusiastic Reiki practitioners have already given me very interesting additional ideas and also increased my understanding of the rules according to which Reiki functions. There have been and continue to be interesting reports of experiences particularly on the topic of Reiki Essences, an application that I have developed for lastingly putting the healing energetic patterns of plants, animals, minerals, or those direct from the subtle world, into a carrier substance like water or sugar by means of a new Second Degree technique. You will find an expressive report by one healing practitioner in the Appendix Two.

In my first three books on the topic of Reiki I have extensively explained the fundamentals of the traditional Usui System of Reiki and also described some interesting new applications as an impulse for the readers' own developments.

The methods introduced in this book are a small[1] but choice excerpt of my research results, which go far beyond the collection of original Reiki methods and knowledge that has been traditionally handed down. This means that this book deals with the avantgarde of Reiki research. In the course of the years, a complex system has developed from this, a system that I call *Rainbow Reiki*. Although Rainbow Reiki is absolutely founded on the Usui System of Reiki and its methods and initiations, it essentially stretches the area of energy work and additionally covers the possibilities of subtle communication. The word "Rainbow" occurred to me because all the colors are contained in the light of the rainbow and this beautiful work of art created by nature has always been seen as a connecting link between heaven and Earth, the human being and the subtle world. Rainbow Reiki is a system of energy work for doing practically anything that can be possibly moved, formed, or developed through energetic effects. And it offers very direct opportunities for contact with the subtle levels of the world, which you will soon see for yourself as you continue to read. Furthermore, I like the sound of this expression. So that's why there's a new term for the higher level of Reiki energy work.

I have tried to compile this method, useful in daily life, in a comprehensively functioning combination that is interesting for both the First and the Second Degree. This experience-based section is supplemented by the necessary theoretical background information, which can help you understand what you are doing and enable you to accept responsibility and deal creatively with Rainbow Reiki. Furthermore, there is a longer section in Chapter One on what I feel to be constructive applications of important ethical fundamentals for

---

[1] A great many things collect in seven years. If I didn't have such an efficient computer, half of my discoveries would certainly have slipped my mind in the meantime. Technology does have its benefits when you get older...

energy work in general and Rainbow Reiki in particular. Without sincere efforts towards personal growth and a fair and wise way of approaching energy work, no genuine spiritual quality of life and no lasting happiness in life can be achieved. This part of the book therefore offers a foundation for holistically understanding Rainbow Reiki. Please read it carefully, listen to your inner voice, and find your own balanced ethical standpoint on the use of energy work, which always should and can be used for the benefit of all participants. Through the living understanding of these basic rules, you will achieve the best results with the Rainbow Reiki methods and easily be able to adapt and develop for your own needs.

One further comment to help you understand the structure of this book: It is quite similar to a hologram in a certain sense. What you read in one chapter is not only useful in the next chapter, but can also be applied to expand and deepen the methods and information of the previous sections. I have presented some of the fundamental techniques and information several times in various places in this book since I wanted to avoid the need for you to page back and forth in order to find the individual components of an exercise from the previous chapters. I hope this won't be too boring for you, simply skip over the repetitions when you have become more experienced with Rainbow Reiki. But some things may be a bit difficult for you to understand the first time you read them. As soon as you have had practical experience on the respective topic and have thought about it for a while, it will become more clear to you. Since this book deals with very advanced methods of Reiki energy work, this means: There's a lot to learn!

I wish you an exciting and insightful time in reading this book. May your experiences with Rainbow Reiki help you achieve self-fulfillment and a life with all the happiness you can stand.

May the power of light and love be with you!

*Walter Lübeck*

11

# CHAPTER ONE

# Fundamentals
# of Rainbow Reiki

As the first step into the colorful world of Rainbow Reiki, let us build a solid foundation for the many experiences and insights that it makes possible. I will give you a survey of the basics of Rainbow Reiki in this chapter. This initially concerns...

## The Usui System of Reiki
## as the Basis for Rainbow Reiki

Rainbow Reiki is based on the traditional Usui System of Reiki. This system of healing by the laying on of hands that is taught through initiations and involves transmitting a special form of subtle, non-polar life energy, Reiki, to be exact, was rediscovered by Dr. Mikao Usui, a Japanese monk, in the writings of an unknown disciple of Buddha while searching for the healing secrets of Jesus Christ and Gautama Buddha in the library of a little Zen monastery at the end of the 19th century. The techniques of energetic healing and the lasting transmission of abilities necessary for this purpose to others were precisely described here. However, the theoretical knowledge of these methods alone wasn't enough to provide Dr. Usui with the ability of working with them in a practical sense. He also had to meditate and fast in a special way at a place of power for 21 days so that he could be connected with the stream of universal life energy, known to us today as Reiki, and thereby became the first Reiki Grand Master of the modern age. He called this method, which he had rediscovered, the *Usui System of Natural Healing* and taught it in all of Japan until about the mid-Twenties. His successor was Dr. Chujiro Hayashi, a medical doctor, who used Reiki in his hospitals for the healing of all types of disorders with great success. The Usui System of Natural Healing came to the West at the end of the Thirties through Hawayo Takata, a student of Hayashi's, who he determined would be his successor as Grand Master. Takata was of Japanese origin and lived as an American citizen on Hawaii. She taught there, as well as on the American continent, in the following decades. She personally trained more than twenty Reiki Masters. When Takata died in 1980, Phyllis Lei Furumoto, who was Takata's granddaughter, and Dr. Barbara Webber-Ray, Takata's close student and friend, took over the office of Grand Master. The two women had different ways of teaching and understanding Reiki, which led to the establishment of two organizations of Reiki Masters that are independent of each other: The Reiki Alliance (Furumoto) and the T.R.T.A.I. (Dr. Webber-Ray). In the following years, Reiki spread with an enormous speed throughout the entire world, and there is probably no country today without at least one Reiki Master. Alone in the German-language region, there are currently, as of May 1994, about 500,000 people who have completed training in the Usui System of Natural Healing and more than 3,000 Reiki Masters who teach it.

What do you absolutely have to learn in the first two degrees in order to use the methods of Rainbow Reiki, the higher level of Reiki, described in this book?[2]

# Preconditions for the Practice of Rainbow Reiki in the First Degree

You must receive four initiations from a traditionally trained Reiki Master[3] within the scope of a seminar on the First Degree, in which the channel for Rainbow Reiki that exists dormant in every person is opened and stabilized for the entire following lifetime. Furthermore, important automatic protective functions against the transmission of healer diseases are established through the initiations of the First Degree. The individual initiations should be a minimum of three hours and a maximum of 24 hours apart in time. The belief in a certain religion, religious community, concept of the world, or way of life is not a prerequisite for initiation into the Reiki methods and their application, no matter which degree is concerned. The same naturally also applies to Rainbow Reiki. In many cases, it is wise to

---

[2] The preconditions listed in the following section are not descriptions of the minimal training contents of the respective Reiki degree, but clarify instead what is absolutely necessary in order to successfully practice the Rainbow Reiki methods described in this book. Moreover, the fundamental Reiki techniques, as well as the important knowledge required for their correct application and further information is described in detail in my books *The Complete Reiki Handbook, Reiki— Way of the Heart*, and *Reiki for First Aid* published by Lotus Light.

[3] I understand a traditionally trained Reiki Master to be someone who has been respectively initiated into all three degrees in the direct physical line of the Grand Masters, starting with Usui, through Hayashi, Takata, Furumoto or Webber-Ray, and the following Masters, and trained in their correct application.

14

let three to four weeks pass after initiation into the First Degree before you learn and experience more of this. Experience has shown that it takes a while for the sometimes intensive healing experiences to be "digested" after becoming involved with the First Degree. In case of doubt, pay attention to what is going on within yourself. You will know when the time is right for you to once again make a journey of discovery.

# Preconditions for the Practice of Rainbow Reiki in the Second Degree

You must receive an initiation into the three symbols and three mantras of the Second Degree through a traditionally trained Reiki Master so that these "tools" can be used within the scope of the Reiki methods for the people concerned. Without an initiation that imparts the power for their application, the symbols and mantras cannot be used for mobilizing and guiding Reiki. Instead, they are simply characters like "A,B,C." The three symbols and the corresponding mantras must be learned by heart so that they are available without any difficulty. You should be familiar with, concretely practice, and be able to use distance treatment, mental healing, and energy intensification without any written "memory aids."

If you have fulfilled these described preconditions in at least the First Degree, you can immediately start with Rainbow Reiki. *In your own interest, please don't assume that the methods depicted in this book work in the described manner if you haven't completed the corresponding Reiki training.*

# According to Which Laws Does Rainbow Reiki Function?

As in every system of energy work, there are also certain laws in the Usui System of Reiki and in Rainbow Reiki, which represents an expansion of the former. Here they are:

1. Reiki is a non-polar force. It is neither yin nor yang. Both hands of a person initiated traditionally into Reiki automatically transmit the same vibration—Reiki, to be precise. This can only be changed by the intensively focussing attention on the conveyance of energies other than Reiki. In this case, these other energies are transmitted in

15

addition to Reiki. The flow of the Reiki force can neither be turned on or off through direct contact.

2. Reiki supports the living processes in everything with which it comes in contact. To the extent that this is permitted, Reiki is drawn in and influences the development of liveliness in a certain physical or mental, emotional, and spiritual area. The more resistance against the development there is, the stronger are the healing reactions that happen. When the brakes of a car take hold, heat and friction occur through the resistance that it offers the movement of the car. The way in which healing reactions are more vehement if a person stubbornly clings to imbalanced structures is comparable.

Within this context, I understand healing reactions in a concrete sense to be:

- Detoxification on physical, psychological, and subtle levels
- Restructuring and the temporary insecurity and/or weakness that it causes
- Increased consumption of energy through frictional losses and re-structuring.[4]

3. Reiki isn't a form of energy capable of *directly* filling out material or energetic deficits or reducing energetic excesses.

4. Reiki is drawn in by the Inner Child/body consciousness of the recipient. For its effect to take place, it isn't necessary that the Reiki practitioner or Reiki recipient consciously believes in the existence or certain effects of Rainbow Reiki.

5. The extent to which Reiki is drawn in depends on how much the Inner Child of the Reiki recipient trusts the practitioner, the situation, and the purpose of developing a new form of behavior triggered by Reiki, a new physical and mental, emotional, and spiritual state, as well as his general need for animating impulses.

6. In order to allow Reiki to have a better effect, it is possible to:
a. Strengthened the flow of the Reiki force through the methods of the Second Degree
b. Direct the Inner Child's attention to the area requiring treatment by way of gentle, soothing touch according to the Metamorphic Method.[5]

---

[4] Also see the corresponding specific literature on the topic of "Healing Reactions" in Appendix Five and compare with the related sections on Chapter Seven.
[5] See Commented Bibliography in Appendix Five.

c. Build a greater feeling of security and a stronger trust in the circumstances and effects of the treatment, as well as in the Reiki practitioner giving treatment

d. Remove from the body of the person being treated the energies or substances that impede his vital processes, or positively change his external circumstances in life, or harmonize in a manner more advantageous to his development the convictions, behavior, emotional blocks, and thought patterns that impede his natural liveliness.

e. Directly provide the individual partial personalities like the Inner Child or the Higher Self with Reiki and consider their views and needs in the developmental work

f. Include the help, advice, and protection from subtle beings with the appropriate special knowledge in the treatment

g. Stimulate processes of perceiving the sense of your own life and the learning steps pending at the present moment.

7. Reiki offers the possibility of subtle communication with the techniques of the Second Degree.

8. Reiki techniques can be used for the indirect guidance of polar energies.

9. The applications of the last two points can be used to a great extent by developing the Reiki practitioner's personality with respect to the ability to love, personal responsibility, and consciousness.

10. Through the direct guidance of the Reiki energy into certain areas of a being's subtle energy system or certain subtle levels, effects can be achieved that are subject to other laws than those of the Reiki energy.

11. The deeper the understanding and acceptance of the laws and areas of effectiveness discussed under point 10, the more extensive and differentiated the energy work of a Reiki practitioner can be.

12. Until the spirit is truly willing to be healed and ready for the necessary changes, the body cannot achieve lasting health and life cannot truly become happy. For this reason: If there is no immediate danger, first heal the spirit.

# What is Healing?

Healing is a concept that summarizes a great many different ideas. This word will be used frequently in this book, and I want to avoid any misunderstandings. I've given a detailed description of it here so that you won't be groping in the dark regarding *my* perspective of healing.

# The Three Steps of Holistic Healing

Holistic development, which I also call healing, occurs in three steps...

### Step 1: Truth

The suppressed or separated material, mental and spiritual, emotional, or energetic aspect that has caused an illness, which I also call an inhibition of development, becomes perceptible and therefore manageable. A constructive confrontation with the underlying imbalance becomes basically possible. Only when this is risked can the next level within the scope of holistic healing take place.

### Step 2: Love

The separated aspect is accepted emotionally, along with the new liveliness. What was previously judged and rejected is now lovingly taken to heart and therefore once again included in a person's own life process.[6] A comprehensive understanding of the problem is not unconditionally necessary for this to happen, but it frequently facilitates the process of learning to accept oneself, which is not exactly easy. Only when this step has been completed can true progress be made. This is also completely possible even if there are still fears and insecurities, as long as these are not suppressed or denied.

### Step 3: Perception

The meaning of the development process and the constructive power of the personality aspect that was split-off or suppressed at one time are so completely integrated that a person's own possibilities for mastering life and/or for development of the self are consid-

---

[6] This makes possible the detoxification processes, as well as the supply of nutrient substances and vibrations.

erably increased. One's very own path in life and the necessary strength to follow it become more conscious, clear, and strong. Life acquires more lightness, meaning, abundance, and joy—no matter what its basic conditions are.

Now that I have presented my perspective of healing and the course of a holistic healing process, I would like to explain what I consider to be the absolutely necessary keystones of spiritual development in greater detail. If a person is involved in a holistic process of development, according to my experience he will develop more extensive abilities in the three topics described below. If the willingness to develop these three qualities is lacking, or if there is a greater imbalance with respect to their acceptance, harmonious growth of the personality, comprehensive physical or mental, emotional, and spiritual healing is not possible.

# The Three Components
## of True Spiritual Development

The path to God is the path of freedom. This doesn't mean freedom from something, but rather freedom for something that brings all of the participants more intensely into the stream of the life force. It helps them develop their uniqueness and contribute to the growth of the beings in their environment. Every true spiritual development can be recognized by these three attributes, explained in greater detail in the following section. You can examine resources and aids for the promotion of your holistic development, such as books, seminars, teachings, and the like, for their suitability on the basis of these three criteria.[7]

### 1. The Ability to Love

The ability to create unity is supported. Hatred, aversion, intolerance, envy, greed, a consciousness of poverty, the helper syndrome, jealousy, hierarchic and competition-oriented thinking, feelings of revenge, denial of one's own needs and physical, emotional, spir-

---

[7] If you take me seriously, which means that you make an effort to create a unity (see under the following point 1) with my thoughts, you won't just simply believe me but will also examine my opinions since I could make a mistake just like anyone else. Just because my opinion appears in print doesn't mean it's right. See under point 2 (Consciousness) and point 3 (Personal Responsibility).

itual, and mental qualities are signs of separation. A person demonstrates the development of the ability to love by increasingly recognizing himself in other beings and things of the Creation, thereby producing a higher degree of unity on the spiritual level. As a result, he will become more satisfied with himself and the world, developing basic trust and a more harmonious ability to relate to others.

## 2. Consciousness

The ability to perceive more of the Creation, to differentiate this perception, and understand the correlations and meaningful concurrence of things in the world is promoted. The development of consciousness is evident in the increased sensitivity and healthier powers of discernment, an expanded understanding of other forms of lifestyles, patience, and devotion to constructive plans that take into consideration the holistic benefit of all participants. A person also supports an intuitive understanding of transpersonal[8] correlations in life.

## 3. Personal Responsibility

Support is given to the ability of accepting more of what affects an individual's own life as being caused on a conscious or unconscious level, and achieving control over it. The development of personal responsibility is shown by the development of trust in your own self and its possibilities. The unique talents hidden within every person become more conscious and can thereby receive more attention. This contributes to everyone's benefit. Through the active satisfaction of your own needs, your personal health will be strengthened and you will achieve more satisfaction, success, creative power, and self-knowledge. A well-developed sense of personal responsibility is the indispensable precondition for the ability to set limits or get involved in every respect.

All three points are absolutely of equal value. One quality can't be developed without the other two. The overriding principle is freely participating in the evolution of the Creation as the realization of the divine will in a way that is satisfying for the individual.

---

[8] Here "transpersonal" means the viewpoint of a situation that goes beyond the moment and the directly perceptible events and correlations. Transpersonal perception is a look behind the scenes of life that permits greater clarity regarding the comprehensive learning processes and problem structures, meaningful possibilities of development, and the concealed developmental inhibitions. Transpersonal insights into the events of everyday life are esoterics put into practice.

# Rainbow Reiki Principles
# for Energy Work and Life Improvement

In order to establish more concrete goals for your energy work and more easily determine the actual success of the efforts, I have established a series of maxims for Rainbow Reiki, some of which are based on rules for living traditionally handed down by the great spiritual currents like Sufism, Taoism, the teaching of Hermes Trismegistos, Shamanism, Zen, and Huna, but have also been influenced in part by my own reflections and experiences.

1. Everything can be found in every other thing and is connected with everything else. Natural individualism doesn't result from the lack of something or the unique existence of certain qualities, but rather through the special emphasis of individual parts of the whole and their unique arrangement, their unmistakable and non-repetitive pattern.

2. Everything is brought into this world through the power of the feminine: new beings, new ideas, energies, as well as the divine force. Because of this, the feminine aspect in everything should be respected, protected, and supported.[9] The greatest feminine force is that of Mother Earth. She is the greatest healer on this level of existence because the energy from the source of life can flow purely and clearly to the sick and needy through her body in order to balance disharmonies in the sense of the cosmic order.

3. Children should be protected from harm and supported in their development to become loving, conscious, and responsibly acting adults. Children are the future.

4. Don't do anything that is unnecessary. Energy and commitment shouldn't be squandered. Do everything necessary so that life can develop in the sense of the cosmic order and organize this as effectively as possible.

---

[9] "Being able to accept," "being open for something," "channeling something into this world" are typical feminine qualities. Perhaps this is why there are so many women and men who are willing to accept their feminine aspect in the Reiki seminars. And perhaps the Reiki initiations and confrontation with this force very much strengthen the feminine, soft, constructive-emotional, and intuitive parts of people who get involved with it.

5. The world appears to you as you are accustomed to perceiving it. If you clear away your filters—the limiting professions of belief, the false concepts of morality, the fears, envy, convictions of inferiority, consciousness of poverty, and similar problems—you can increasingly perceive what the true world is made of. The result will be that you can better deal with life when you have integrated these perceptions into your personality.

6. A person who can let go can also accept. A person who can say "no" can also say "yes."

7. Love expresses itself in life-affirming behavior and the joy of being together with other parts of the Creation.

8. Life energy flows towards the attention of the Inner Child/body consciousness.

9. Without devotion, there would be no power; without service, no ruling.

10. Anger, pain, and fear are exhortations to harmonize the life process more closely with your own genuine needs.

11. Spirituality grows when you understand and emotionally integrate practical experiences.

12. What separates makes sick. What unites heals.

13. Loving joy in life is the power that brings a person closer to God.

14. The subtle forces can't help you if you don't ask them for help. They respect the freedom of all beings.

15. Respect and gratefulness dissolve separation and invite unity.

16. Emotional energies can only be expressed through the body. Otherwise, new blocks or mechanisms of repression are created.

17. Music, dance, and singing that are oriented towards the vibrations of the natural life forces open the hearts of people who devote themselves to God and His helping power. If nothing helps anymore and Reiki is not accepted by the Inner Child, this resource can still effect a resolution of the block and support acceptance of the healing Reiki energy.

# Responsibility—An Important Topic in Relation to Rainbow Reiki

You will become familiar with a great many highly effective methods of energy work in this book and, with a bit of practice, be capable of doing things that people without Reiki experience probably think are possible only in dreams. The Rainbow Reiki methods are meant to heal you and others in the spiritual sense, to support the growth of the personality, and make possible a friendly, loving cooperation with beings of the subtle worlds: the devas, angels, and natural forces.

I feel it is very important that as many people as possible who are initiated into Reiki use this significant knowledge in a meaningful way because our world and its many different inhabitants urgently need more support in these difficult times as the Age of Pisces fades out and the Age of Aquarius is beginning to dawn. It would help all of us if the Rainbow Reiki knowledge is used in a responsible manner. There would be many problems if people exploit Rainbow Reiki with egotistic motives, showing disrespect for the freedom of others, arrogance, or a striving for power. I have thought about this a great deal and talked with my spiritual teachers about this topic time and again before making the decision to write this book, which means no longer imparting the fundamentals of Rainbow Reiki solely in direct contact from teacher to student. The decision was ultimately mine, and as you can see, it was "pro." I could never have reached so many people through seminars and lectures as through this book. And I have the strong feeling that time is slowly running out for a successful restructuring of our society and lifestyle in the holistic sense.

I therefore ask you to carefully examine your motives for involvement with energy work in general and Rainbow Reiki in particular time and again, acting for the holistic benefit of all participants to the best of your ability. This effort alone is already a wonderful path of personality training and you will also support social evolution, setting a good example for others that will stimulate them to reflect and look inside themselves.

It naturally isn't possible to always do the right thing since human beings sometimes do make mistakes, have a bad day, or simply just don't know enough. Because of this, I will now give you an opportunity to once and for all side with the active promoters of the divine stream of life and make sure that you will receive extensive help from the powers of love and light. For this purpose I use the *Light Vow Ritual*. Take the time to read it and if you really want to do this of your own free will, carry it out. It will give you protection, loving care, and help that you can always rely on. It is an initiation in the sense of the conscious decision to actively and lastingly support the good forces of the universe. God only has our hands on this level of existence, and if we decide to work together with Him for the good of the development of his Creation, we will contribute much to increasingly bringing his vibration back into this world and changing things for the better.

# The Light Vow Ritual

Set aside a good hour of your time to do this. Fill the bathtub and perfume the water with a few drops of sandalwood oil of a natural origin. Take a bath, thoroughly and consciously washing yourself. Perceive the water and the fragrance of the oil. Surrender to the relaxation and enjoy the pleasant warmth around you. When you wash yourself, become aware that you are leaving the things of everyday life behind you and removing disruptive vibrations from your aura.[10] Rinse yourself off with lukewarm water at the end. Then wrap yourself in a comfortable bathrobe, take a blanket, and look for a room in which you can remain undisturbed for a while. Stand with bare feet, legs about one-and-a-half shoulder-widths apart. Lift your arms to the heavens, bend your knees somewhat, and raise your face a bit. Perceive the ground beneath your feet, which always securely supports you and permits the feeling that you are in unity with other parts of the Creation. Remain with this feeling for a few breaths. Then direct your attention to the sky above the top of your head, from which life energies constantly flow into you in and attempt to support your development. Also perceive the contact with these energies for a few breath cycles. Now direct your attention to the flow of your breath. Each time you inhale, visualize the light stream of heavenly energy that flows into you through the top of your head and fills your body from head to foot.

Every time you exhale, let a stream of dark Earth energy flow into you through your feet and fill you completely. Repeat this breathing exercise slowly and consciously for at least thirty times. It balances your body energies and helps you come into contact with your Inner Child.[11] Now stand up straight and light three candles—a light-colored

---

[10] For this ritual to be effective, it isn't necessary for you to *believe* in its effectiveness. Be open for the experience and carry it out as stated, then it will function as described.

[11] The *Inner Child* is an active part of your personality that usually is unconscious and independent from the rest of your mind in broad areas. It is responsible for feelings, active and passive energy work, vitality, and holistic thinking. It doesn't understand the language of the analytic, rational consciousness. Its methods of communication include rituals, sensual impressions, and the like. You will find more on this topic in almost every chapter, particularly Chapter Four.

one for your Higher Self[12], a dark one for your Inner Child, and a violet one for the conscious, rational part of your personality, your Middle Self. Now you just need to light some sandalwood incense, the aroma of which will relax you and foster the communication with your Inner Child—then the concluding portion of the ritual can begin: preparing and signing a contract with yourself and the powers of light and love.

Take a blank piece of paper, perhaps handmade paper, in order to also optically highlight the significance of this document. Please write with violet ink or a pen with a violet color. When everything is ready, put your hands on your lap for a moment, close your eyes, feel how you are breathing, and say quietly: "I am at my center, I am with myself and will now enter into a new, wonderful phase of my life through my clear and distinct decision!"

Now take the paper and pen and write:

---

## *My Light Vow*

I,_____ (your complete name),

born on _____ at _____ (time, if known),

in _____(place),

irrevocably and of my free will declare herewith that I will use all the spiritual powers to which I gain access only for the best of all those involved. I will respect the freedom of all beings when I put these abilities to use and only do so with their consent in relation to them. I call you, you high powers of light and love, to be witnesses and guardians of this contract and ask you to support me in my efforts, to help me when I need help, and to advise me when I need advice in order to fulfill my intention in life.

I hereby irrevocably dedicate my spiritual development to the universal powers of light and love and gratefully and respectfully accept their protection and care.

_____

(Place, date) (signature)

---

[12] Your *Higher Self* is also a largely independent portion of the overall personality and, among other things, is responsible for the fulfillment of your life plan. This means you have the experiences in this world and in this incarnation that you selected for yourself before your birth as comprehensive learning themes. There will be more about this in the following chapter, particularly in Chapter Four.

It is also wonderful to take the Light Vow in a group of like-minded friends. This transformational ritual only needs to be done once, but it's so beautiful that I repeat it with almost every seminar group that I teach in aura-reading or the advanced levels of Rainbow Reiki. In addition to the connection with the powers of light and love, it's an effective spiritual purification method that can be carried out on special occasions with great benefit for the progress of spiritual development.

Now you have become a bit more familiar with the fundamentals of Rainbow Reiki and can already start with the first practical experiences.

## A Little Learning Tip for You...

The exercises explained in the following chapters are sometimes a bit long. Make it easier for yourself to learn them by reading the instructions written for them onto a cassette at a slow tempo with the corresponding pauses. Play this when you practice as long as you are still uncertain about it. This method has often helped me learn longer procedures. Don't let the technology bother you. It doesn't just have disadvantages. As soon as you know the respective exercise by heart, then you'll no longer need the "prompter." If you can learn the Rainbow Reiki methods in a group with others, let one member of the group read the respective exercise slowly and with the pauses while the others carry it out.

*When a person is happy, he can make others happy.*
*If he does this, he encreases his own happiness.*

(Johann Ludwig Wilhelm Gleim)

CHAPTER TWO

# Aura and Chakra Work
# with Rainbow Reiki

As an introduction to practical energy work with Rainbow Reiki, here are some methods that can be applied with the tools of the First Degree. You can make some of them even more effective with the help of the Second Degree techniques. When this is the case, I have also explained the corresponding procedure.

## How You Can Deal with
## Healing Reactions...

Take your time in reading this chapter and then allow enough time for each exercise in order to learn it and experience its deep effects. Don't overdo it by trying out everything or too much at one time. The applications presented here will in no way harm you if you carry them out precisely as they are described here and if you aren't suffering from any serious physical, emotional, or mental illness.[13] However, you can get an energy hangover or vehement healing reactions to the development-promoting contact with Rainbow Reiki.

After every exercise, take the time to walk for half an hour and simply be with yourself in order to ground the energies released from the blocks and calmly integrate what might have come up. Another possibility is having something light to eat afterwards, to paint what you have felt, or dance to express what has moved you and thereby constructively translate it into action. Then you can let go of it. In no case should you start the Rainbow Reiki energy work when you are very stressed, under pressure to produce results, or in a hurry. Stress considerably reduces the control of the subtle abilities, as well as reducing the flow of subtle energies.

---

[13] If you are seriously ill, you certainly shouldn't carry out any unusual vital-energy exercises and doctor around on yourself. Instead, have yourself attended to by a doctor who works holistically and only use other healing methods in consultation with him until you have regained your strength and are healthy once again!

If you have friends with a similar approach to life, then you can start a Rainbow Reiki self-discovery group with them. The exercises are particularly fun to do and much easier to learn when you're not alone.

If headaches, dizziness, a feeling of unreality, or any other oppressive sensations occur during or after an exercise, as long as it was correctly carried out this is often because of the energies that have been released from the dissolved or fully harmonized blocks in the person treated. They can't yet find their place since other blocks are obstructing their path to the fields of activity appropriate for them. You can help them become integrated into the energy structure in the right way by treating the upper area of the soles of your client's feet for several minutes. In difficult cases, alternately provide the foot soles and the navel area directly with Reiki and have your partner breath into the hara. This is a switching point for vital energy, not a chakra, found about two fingers beneath the navel on the central line of the body. After the symptoms have receded, don't forget to do the grounding exercises mentioned above, going for a walk, dancing, eating, and the like.

A further method of harmonization is the so-called "chakra balance," a standard technique of the First Degree course. To do this, provide the 1st and 6th chakras, then the 2nd and 5th, and finally the 3rd and 4th with Reiki, each pair for about three minutes. If you are initiated into the Second Degree, you can also give a mental healing with the constantly repeated suggestion of "energy balance." If the described reactions occur on a regular basis, the affected person should no longer participate in energy work until he has been examined by a competent doctor who uses holistic methods in order to clarify the causes of the overreaction.

# How You as a Practitioner Can Deal with Imbalances That You Take On from Your Clients

As a practitioner, you should thoroughly wash your hands with soap, up to above the wrists, before and after each session of energy work. Both you and the person to be treated should remove all watches, rings, and chains before the exercise. If you have taken symptoms of disruptive energy patterns into your aura from a client, shower thoroughly, using lukewarm water for some of the time. If you frequently take on other people's symptoms, clarify why you want to suffer and change this into the lasting wish of wanting to feel well. This conviction will take some time in order to be completely integrated into the personality and represents a large step in your development. Practice setting better limits on the emotional level and find out why you haven't wanted to do this up to now. Strengthen yourself by clearly reducing your stress level, eating healthier foods, getting enough sleep, establishing a more regular rhythm in life for yourself, doing more fitness sports (in no case should these be performance-oriented!), and satisfying your other physical needs. In addition, strengthen your 1st, 3rd, and 5th chakras with Reiki and the appropriate healing stones and make sure that you become more stable emotionally. Give some thought to how you can put the spiritual principle of "personal responsibility" into practice.

Because of the Reiki initiations, there is no way that imbalances outside energies can get into your own inner energy system during a treatment situation, entrench themselves and cause the so-called healer diseases. This is one of Reiki's very great advantages. However, the perception of outside energies continues as before and can be very irritating if you don't make sure that the vibrational pattern causing this disappears from your aura (the outer energy system responsible for communication with others) or that you no longer hold onto it. Everything that promotes the natural flow of the aura from the inside to the outside, strengthening and stabilizing its structure through personal growth, will help you better cope with coming into contact with imbalanced energies.

The rules discussed in this section correspondingly apply to the entire book and are basically valid for every type of Reiki energy work. So let's get down to the practice!

## Exercise I:
### *Chakra development with the Reiki Powerball*

I came across the Reiki powerball technique while searching for a more simple, intensive, yet still gentle method of chakra work that can also reach and harmonize the deeper levels of an energy center. Other methods have a hard time going beyond the relatively superficial areas of a chakra in their effects and temporarily create a fair amount of disorder in the process or they can only be successfully applied by people who have a great deal of experience. The Reiki powerball technique has proved itself to be quite successful up to now. Even extensive blocks are usually not an obstacle for it. And if you simply want to have more "power" for yourself, for example, after work or training or any other energy-eaters, the Reiki powerball is practically unbeatable. Oh, yes—if you want to do something good for your plants or healing stones, you can also try out this technique on them. If you need a compress that is intensively charged with Reiki for bruises, headache, stomachache, nausea, or wounds, then use the Reiki powerball technique to impregnate a handkerchief, bandage, or the like. Water, oils, and ointments can also be charged strongly in a simple and quick manner. You will quickly discover many other applications yourself if you experiment with the Reiki powerball.

### Step 1: Creating the Reiki Powerball

Before the powerball can develop its effect on other people and objects, you must first create it. To do this, hold your hands, palms facing each other, about 20 to 30 centimeters apart at the level of your heart and about 30 centimeters from your body. Wait a moment and feel your way into the energy that increasingly collects between your hands. Now gently move them back and forth, like grass swaying in the wind. Change the distance between them somewhat while you do this. First in one direction, then the other. Feel how the power continues to grow. Feel the resistance of the Reiki powerball when you move your hands a bit closer to each other. Perceive how your hands are gently held back by the energy when you slowly pull them away from each other. During the entire exercise, be sure that the

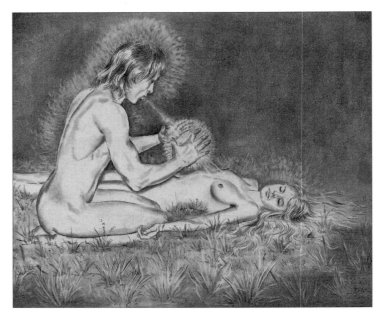

*The Reiki Powerball—a new form of chakra therapy*

palms of your hands always remain facing each other, that they don't touch each other, but also that there is no more than a distance of about 40 centimeters between them.

### *Step 2: Application of the Reiki Powerball*
### Variation A:

Continue to hold your hands with the insides turned towards each other, about 20 to 30 centimeters apart from each other. In this position, move them to a distance of about 30 centimeters from each other in front of one of your exercise partner's six lower major chakras.[14] Now blow gently and constantly through your hands to the corresponding chakra until you have exhaled completely. Repeat this process—the blowing—at least two more times. If you haven't had much experience with this exercise and/or the way your exercise partner reacts to it, then don't blow more than six or seven times. While doing this, direct your attention to the energy that you move through the power of your breath and the effect it has in the chakra to which you are directing it. After each time you blow the energy into the chakra, ask your partner about his perceptions. If some sort of strong imbalance becomes perceptible and doesn't disappear on its own after a few minutes, help him ground himself by carrying out some of the exercises described at the beginning of the chapter with him.

### Variation B:

Slowly move the Reiki powerball as close as possible to exercise partner's corresponding chakra by guiding your hands in this direction. During the first attempts with this method, don't establish the contact for more than about 30 seconds. Ask your partner to keep you informed about his perceptions. If necessary, ground him. You can also use the Reiki powerball by putting your hands on the appropriate spot, approaching it from the narrow side of the body. Then move the energy ball into the body by holding one hand on the front of the body and the other on the back of your partner's body. The insides of the hands must naturally face each other the whole time. Moving the hands gently back-and-forth is helpful in maintaining the powerball.

---

[14] You should only work with the 7th chakra, the crown energy center, when you have had enough experience in dealing with energy work in general and this exercise in particular. Otherwise, it could be too intensive when larger blocks obstruct the released energy from flowing out of the head area, creating an imbalance by the one-sided, non-grounded dissolution of subtle congestion. By the way, it isn't really necessary to work with the 7th chakra since its condition results from the functioning of the lower 6 major chakras. If they are in good shape, then the crown chakra will also be in order. Things don't work quite as easily in the opposite direction.

**Please note**: If you move your hands apart at some point in order to do something else with them, for example, to treat your client's feet or do chakra balancing, you have to recreate the Reiki powerball each time before you can work with it again!

*The effect of this exercise:* A large amount of concentrated Reiki energy collects between your hands as a result of this exercise. The breath has a special quality that strongly supports the impact and reception of subtle energies in the human energy system, particularly in the chakras. The chakra provided with Reiki in this manner can more easily free itself of blocks that impede its natural function and more quickly balance a possible charging deficit or release an excess of energy. Most people feel refreshed, strengthened, centered, and more relaxed after a treatment with the Reiki powerball.

## Exercise II:
### *Opening chakras to make deeper-reaching developmental work possible—Closing chakras to protect the growth process from disruptive outside influences*

In order for every type of chakra work with Reiki to have an even better, more lasting, and more gentle effect, the respective energy center can be opened before an application. When this has been done, it is *absolutely* necessary to close the chakra once again. Within this context, the "opening" of a chakra doesn't mean an expansion of its function in a qualitative or quantitative sense, but solely the creation of an intensified state of acceptance for outside influences of all types. "Closing" also doesn't mean a qualitative or quantitative limitation, but rather solely creating a state of natural protection from every type of disruptive outside influence, which in no way impedes the normal communication of the energy center. Instead, it makes this and the chakra's healthy functioning possible in the first place.

### *How to Open a Chakra*

*Step 1*: Establish contact with the respective energy center by concentrating your attention on it and holding one hand—it doesn't matter which—about 10 to 15 centimeters above it, with the palm turned towards the chakra. You will feel an intensified flow, a sensation of "being drawn towards" it, more warmth, a feeling of familiarity, or perhaps even a pulsation when the connection between your hands and the structure of the chakra has been established.

**Step 2**: Slowly, consciously, and gently move your hand counter-clockwise in three circles above the chakra. At the same time, formulate the wish for it to open and imagine, for example, a blossom that unfolds a bit more with each circular movement of your hand and is completely open when the third circle has been completed. Feel the change in the vibration of the energy center.

**Step 3**: Charge the energy center by holding one or both hands above it, moving in a slight horizontal and vertical direction, as if swinging in the wind. If you are initiated into the Second Degree, use the sign for energy intensification and the corresponding mantra to amplify the flow of the Reiki power. Further possibilities of energy work can naturally also be used within this step. For example, gemstones (purify beforehand!) can be put on the chakra or chakra oils massaged into it. In any case, always be very gentle with a chakra in an opened state. If the session is interrupted for any reason, always carefully close each opened energy center before doing anything else!

### How to Close a Chakra

**Step 1**: As explained in Step 1 for opening a chakra.

**Step 2**: Slowly, consciously, and gently move your hand that is in contact with the energy center clockwise in three complete circles above the chakra. At the same time, formulate the wish in your mind for it to close and create a blossom in front of your inner eye that closes more and more until it is completely closed when your hand has completed the third circle. Then give the chakra a moment of Reiki. If necessary, ground your client's energies by giving Reiki to the soles of his feet. When doing so, instruct him to breath calmly and evenly into his lower belly.

After a session in which you have worked with a chakra in an open state, it is highly recommended that the person treated take a nap of 15 to 20 minutes!

## Exercise III:
### "Twisting out" energy blocks and what to observe when you do this

When you attune yourself very much to a client during intensive aura or chakra work, it can happen that you notice energetic blocks on the surface of an energy center or in the energy field around the body. It may be a type of shadow or a zone in which your hands are restrained in their movement, where things are "tough" somehow. You can dissolve this congested energy through the following technique and thereby help the body make space for a lively flow of the forces.

*Step 1*: Stretch out one hand and hold it so that the fingertips are in the area of the blocked energy. Wait a moment and attune to it by simply at the same time keeping your attention on the congestion and your hand. Then move your hand, first slowly and then increasingly quickly, clockwise and about 50 centimeters away from your client. Shake off the energy into the Earth, which will integrate it into the natural flow of the forces. Repeat this process until you no longer perceive any congestion in this part of the energy field. Then hold both your hands over this area for about one or two minutes with the palms facing your partner.

If you are initiated into the Second Degree, repeatedly use the intensification symbol and corresponding mantra. Slightly move your hands back and forth in a horizontal and vertical direction, as if they were dancing in the wind. This causes the energy field to be charged and stabilized at the point where the block was and where an amount of energy, which is often considerable, has been directed out of it. If you don't recharge this area with fresh vibrations, new imbalances could easily arise and outside energies enter, entrench themselves, and have negative effects on the respective person. At the end of a session, your client should carry out the following little exercise, which also functions when a person hasn't been initiated into a Reiki degree: Put the right hand on the heart chakra and the left hand on the solar plexus chakra. Pay attention to what's going on inside for a moment. Then say out loud: "I thank the energies that have left me for their participation in my life process and wish for them to go where they bring blessings." Once again pay attention to what is happening inside, and then remove the hands from the energy center. If this exercise is carried out in a serious manner, new blocks won't take the place of the old ones that have been directed away from it.

If more than three blocks have been twisted out during a session, about three minutes of Reiki should be given to the heart chakra and solar plexus chakra at the end of the treatment. Also treat the soles of the feet.

# Exercise IV:
## *Systematic aura massage with Reiki*

### *Step 1: Clearing the aura*

The client stretches out on his back. He shouldn't cross his legs. Instead, spread them a bit. The arms lie relaxed next to the body, with some distance between. The practitioner now holds his hand over the heart chakra and the hara at a distance of about 10 to 15 centimeters from the client's body[15], closes his eyes, and directs his attention to what's going on inside the other person.

This part of the technique results in an adaptation of both people's aura-field vibrations, which enormously facilitates effective, smooth energy work of any type. After several minutes or when the practitioner feels a sort of acceptance or resonance with the other person, he changes his hands (still without making any direct physical contact with the client's body) over to two positions to the right and left of the center of the body, directly under the collarbone and above the breasts. To intensify the effect, your hands can gently move a bit in the horizontal and vertical directions, as you learned in the first exercise for the Reiki powerball.

After about five minutes, the hands are placed above the top of the head. First sense this area for a moment, then do gentle, stroking movements on one arm down beyond the hand and then on the other arm in the same manner. If the practitioner's hands are then led back to the top of the head, a distance of about 50 centimeters should be maintained from the body. When stroking downwards, go back to a distance of about 10 to 15 centimeters. Stroke through the energy field of each arm five to ten times in this way. This portion of the exercise clears the client's aura and promotes the effectiveness of any treatment that follows. The ability of the hands for subtle perception can also be intensified in this way.

Now place the hands above the top of the head and stroke just to the right and left of the body's midline[16], down to around the respective middle of both thighs. Repeat this five to ten times. Then position the hands to the right and left above each hipbone and calmly feel the vibrations there for a moment. In closing, smooth out each leg from this point to distinctly beyond the foot. When bringing the hands back to the starting position above the hipbones, be sure to maintain a distance of about 50 centimeters in order to not disturb the flow of the aura.

---

[15] Maintain this distance of the practitioner's hands to the client's body for the entire session. No body contact takes place during this exercise.

[16] By midline of the body I mean the straight line existing between the tip of the nose and the navel, as well as its extension upwards and downwards.

After the aura has been thoroughly cleared and stabilized in this manner, three important energy centers are activated in order to give the harmonious state of the aura fields a greater stability. To do this, the middle finger of one hand, it doesn't matter which hand since the same type of energy, namely Reiki, flows in both of them, should at first carefully and slowly approach the 6th chakra and hold still about one finger above it for a moment, then pull away just as carefully and slowly. Next, repeat the same process at the heart chakra and then the 2nd chakra. Afterwards, treat the soles of the feet for about 5 minutes if this step is used without the following step.

All your movements should take place in a very calm, conscious, and careful manner. If no further energy work is to be done, the client should rest for at least 15 minutes after completion of this exercise. Important restructuring of the energy system takes place during this time if the body and mind are not immediately burdened with demands. Even alone, this first step of the entire exercise is a highly effective technique of aura work and can be meaningfully applied on its own without any further measures.

### Step 2: Dynamization of the aura

This step should only take place after the first step, explained directly above. Otherwise, the technique won't have a reliable effect! Once again, as in the entire process, a distance of 10 to 15 centimeters away from the body is maintained and the work is done in a calm, conscious, and careful manner.

The practitioner positions his hands just below the client's feet for a moment. During this time, feel your way into the flow of energy there. Then, with strokes of about 20 centimeters, first stroke over one leg, then the other, up to the area of the navel. Each leg should receive this treatment no more than three times. Be sure to maintain a distance of about 50 centimeters from the surface of the body when moving the hands back to their starting position.

When this portion of the exercise has been completed, hold the hands above the lower belly for a time and feel the energy there. From here, stroke just right and left of the body midline up to the chest. Again hold the hands above the heart area and perceive the energy there. Continue to stroke upwards, first over the one shoulder and the arm down to the hand (but not beyond it), and then do the same for the other shoulder and hand. Move the hands back to the heart chakra, feel the energy there for a moment, and then end the exercise by gently stroking up to the hairline.

A rest of 15 minutes is also recommended afterwards here.

This exercise brings "fresh wind" into the aura, intensively charging it with the healing Earth energy and Reiki. The channels responsible for the direction of the Earth forces into a person's center are purified and stabilized.

## Exercise V:
### *Simple, channeled Reiki-aura/chakra work*

The practitioner places his hands over the client's heart chakra, with the palms turned towards the latter, about 10 to 15 centimeters above the client's body. The practitioner's arms must remain relaxed and free while doing this. After some time, the arms begin to move on their own. They will swing back and forth, more or less in large circles, ellipses, and lines. The practitioner shouldn't consciously cause or try to control these movements! Simply let it happen and follow the arms and hands with your body if they want to go to areas of the client's body that are far removed from the starting area. Vertical movements are also possible. The treatment is complete when your arms stop moving. Afterwards, the hands should be held still above the 3rd and 4th chakras at a distance of about 10 to 15 centimeters for at least three minutes. Then slowly move the hands away from this point. If the treatment must be interrupted for any reason whatsoever before the arms stop moving on their own, the soles of the client's feet must be provided with Reiki for about three additional minutes.

A rest of at least 15 minutes is recommended afterwards.

This exercise is based on the abilities of the Inner Child to directly perceive and control subtle flows of energy. The Inner Child is present in every human being, usually as a subconscious portion of the personality. You will learn more about its attributes and abilities in the following chapters, particularly in the fourth. The Inner Child is practically a specialist for energy work. But it can only become active when the conscious, rationally working personality portion can bring itself to give up control for a time. Then phenomena occur, such as those described in this exercise, which can be put to meaningful use. In the process, the Inner Child disentangles the blocked energies in the fields of the aura and helps reestablish their natural flow. The rational mind could never do this in such a differentiated way like the Inner Child since the latter moves within its own world while doing so and immediately translates its subtle perceptions into active energy work, without the censorship of the intellectual apparatus (which is ponderous in this respect). Try out this type of aura work. You will learn to love it because of its elegance and effectiveness. At the same time, you will achieve increasingly good contact with your Inner Child the more you work with it.

# Exercise VI:
## *Direct cooperation with the Inner Child and Higher Self to make aura and chakra energy work more intensive*

This exercise will be something special for you if you've been initiated into the Second Degree. The last exercise described above can even be improved if, before beginning, you create a type of "standing line" to your Inner Child and your Higher Self through the distance contact as per the Second Degree. This is how it goes:

Use the symbol for distance treatment and the symbol for energy intensification, as well as the corresponding mantras. Turn your hands away from yourself and assume that your Inner Child will be somewhere around where they are directed. Don't try to somehow imagine it for yourself! Say out loud, or in your thoughts, three times: "Inner Child of (add your first and last name)." Use the intensification symbol and the corresponding mantra a few more times in order to intensify the flow of Reiki. If an image shows up on its own, that's all right. But it isn't important for the success of this exercise.

Repeat the same process, but this time after the initial use of the necessary symbols and mantras, direct the flow of the Reiki energy by saying out loud, or thinking, three times: "Higher Self of (add your first and last name)." Also intensify the flow of energy several times here. In any case, don't try to imagine your Higher Self while you do this. If it shows itself in one form or another, this is fine. But it isn't necessary for the success of this exercise.

Then request that your Inner Child and your Higher Self participate in the following aura/chakra work. Always treat these two portions of the personality with respect and attention! Wait another moment, and then proceed as described in Exercise V. When you have completely finished the treatment, always take leave from any distance contact in the same way you learned in the basic Second Degree course and carefully end it.

Before you carry out the exercise explained in this section, establish contact with your Inner Child and your Higher Self individually several times for 2 to 3 minutes in order to get used to them. At the beginning, you shouldn't do this more often than two or three times a week. If you manage well with it, then establish contact with them as often and for as long as you like. Now you can also cooperate with them in the aura/chakra work.

# Rainbow Reiki Mandalas Healing Patterns That Help Bring Light and Love to the Earth

Rainbow Reiki Mandalas are a new method for creating a lasting effect through the unique combination of high-intensity and high-quality vibrations that harmonize material and subtle energetic elements. Rainbow Reiki Mandalas function like converging lens for spiritual energy streams of all types. The possibilities for their application are almost limitless. With them, you can create personal places of power, make healing water, engage in many different types of energy work, purify rooms and give them a lasting pleasant atmosphere that supports relaxing, healing, learning, or sensuality, for example. Your garden or other places in nature can become more inviting for subtle helping forces through such patterns. The aura of special mandalas can make it clear to pests that they are not needed, help plants to grow better, assist in reducing environmental damage by the activating the natural purifying powers and contributing to the harmonization of the Earth. Even the act of setting up a Rainbow Reiki Mandala is a meditative process for the person who does it, enormously increasing and clarifying the vibrations of his energy body for at least some amount of time.

## The Story of the Rainbow Reiki Mandala Method's Origin

While searching for ways of permitting healing subtle powers to have an effect without the necessity of a person's constant presence, I found something in old Druid writings about working together with nature beings through patterns of plants parts and healing stones that are made according to a certain ritual. Unfortunately, for an inexperienced person the preparation for this method was very lengthy and it wasn't possible to make anything with a meaningful effect from the given materials except for a work of art that was nice to look at. Yet, after a number of experiments I found this way of approaching the forces of the spiritual level to be so wonderful and effective that I swore I would find a feasible way, at least for every person who has been initiated into the First Reiki Degree, to use the healing patterns.

Through a teacher, I learned an ancient power song from the Polynesian region that has a very useful effect in a simple manner: it invites the creative forces to participate in whatever is being done at the particular moment. I tried out this mantra in chakra energy work, room purifications, and for charging water and healing stones. It had a fantastic effect, and many of my students now work with it in the meantime. I combined this song with the possibilities of the First Degree and my shamanistic knowledge. First I carefully tried out this new way of making patterns, which can bring subtle forces into our world, alone and then together with my advanced students. It worked beautifully! This was the birth of the Rainbow Reiki Mandala method, making the old knowledge of the wise Druids available once again to many people. I wish you much enjoyment in trying it out!

# Hey Loa, Key Loa, Manaho Lo
## An Old Healing Song
## and Its Various Effects

First, it is necessary for you to become familiar with the healing song mentioned above. You should be able to sing it, both lyrics and melody, by heart.

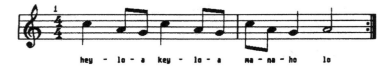

hey - lo - a  key - lo - a  na - na - ho  lo

When you have learned the song, you can start working with the Rainbow Reiki Mandalas. These patterns can basically be created with plants parts, rocks, or crystals.

# Rainbow Reiki Plants Mandalas

**Step 1:** Exactly define, at best in writing, the purpose for which you want to lay a Rainbow Reiki mandala.

**Step 2:** Go to a forest, park, a familiar power place[17], or your yard. Take some time to feel what is taking place there and the flows of energy at this spot. Touch the Earth for several minutes with the palms of your hands and give it Reiki. Give yourself Reiki for about five minutes and sing this song for the subtle helper forces of this place at least nine times while doing so: "Hey loa, key loa, manaho lo." It doesn't hurt to do it even more often and is beneficial for you and the beings of nature. Afterwards, remain in this position and request that the natural forces accept, protect, and guide you. Ex-

---

[17] Compare with Chapter Five of this book.

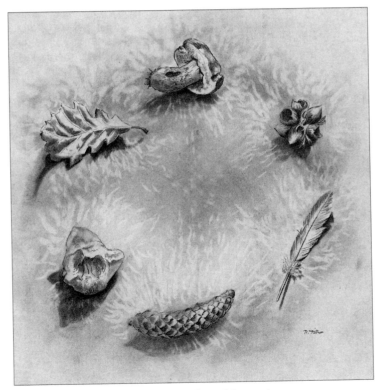

*Rainbow Reiki plant mandalas collect healing subtle energies*

plain what you plan to do—for example, that you would like to have a pattern for general healing purposes or one to help your child sleep better and overcome his fears, or one to harmonize certain Earth rays (please think of the place where these occur when doing this) so that they know what they can do for you. In exchange for their help, offer them Reiki and the song (see below).

Then let yourself intuitively be guided, without thinking about it, to the appropriate plant parts (and sometimes complementary stones and feathers) that the guardians of this place consider suitable for the Rainbow Reiki Mandala. Give each object Reiki for some time before you pick it up and sing the "Hey loa, key loa..." song at least nine times while you do this. Offer thanks for what has been given to you, carefully pick up the object, and stow it in a bag that you use only for collecting power objects for Rainbow Reiki Mandalas. You should either buy this bag new or make it yourself. It must be made of natural materials. Before you use it for the first time, give it Reiki for at least 10 minutes in order to purify it and bring it into contact with the universal flow of energy by singing the "Hey loa, key loa..." song in order to consecrate it. Take only plant parts that are no longer on living plants! Don't tear or cut anything off of a living plant! When you have collected everything, take leave of the forces of nature and your subtle helpers, thank them once again, put your hands on the Earth for a while and give it Reiki. End this part of the work by letting Reiki flow to your heart and your solar plexus for about five minutes. If you feel like it, sing the healing song for the nature beings a few times.

**Step 3:** Go to the place where you would like to lay out the Rainbow Reiki Mandala. Be sure that you are undisturbed there, and attune yourself to it for a few minutes. At the same time, give yourself Reiki on your heart and forehead chakra. Then spread out all the objects next to you, give them Reiki for a moment, and feel your way into the vibrations that they are sending out. Think about your plans, ask the powers of light and love for guidance, and carefully pick up all the pieces. Hold them in both hands in front of your heart, give them Reiki, and look at them as if they were a person you love. While doing so, sing the mantra "Hey loa, key loa..." nine times. Then hold the objects up to the heavens, look at them with a loving gaze, and also sing the mantra nine times here and give them Reiki. Pause for a moment and perceive the strong, clear power now emanating from the consecrated pieces. Start to sing the song again and continue until the ritual is finished. One after the other, carefully put each object onto the spot where you want to create the mandala. Put each down one after the other so that they are *right* in the way they lay on or next to each other. Be sure that the distances between them and the angles are correct. You will feel it when everything is *right*. Perceive how the vibrations become stronger with every piece you lay down. Trust the guidance by the powers of light and love and don't let your intellect get involved. It can't help you with this type of work, it can't even really understand it.

When you have laid down everything, wait for a moment, put both hands on the area of your heart, and thank the powers of light and love. Feel the power of the Rainbow Reiki Mandala, which is now fully capable of functioning. Now it is working and ready to help and to heal.

**Step 4:** When you want to undo the pattern, proceed as follows:
Attune yourself with the Rainbow Reiki Mandala for a moment by putting one hand on your forehead and the other on your heart, looking at it, and opening yourself for its power. Thank it for its services, bow to it, and carefully pick up every object. When you have them all in your hands, thank the powers of light and love and the heavens and the Earth for their support. Stow everything away carefully in the bag prepared for this purpose.

In contrast to the crystal patterns described later, the plant patterns are not suitable for being collected after the work has been done. Use them for purposes in which they can remain unchanged in one place for a longer period of time. Otherwise, they will easily fall apart. If you would like to give them more stability, press them into wet clay in order to fix them in place and then let it dry in the air. You can naturally also do this with Rainbow Reiki Crystal Mandalas, for example, when they are to be worn as an amulet or when you want to move them from one place to another in a single piece.

Whether you lay out plant patterns or crystal patterns for a certain purpose is up to your personal taste. When in doubt, let yourself be advised by an old power place.[18] They have also taught me much about such work.

# Rainbow Reiki Crystal Mandalas

You can also lay Rainbow Reiki Mandalas with all types of healing stones and crystals. You can actually use any stone for this purpose. If you are knowledgeable about the effects of various types of healing stones, choose those suitable for your respective plans. The Rainbow Reiki Mandala method will qualitatively expand its spe-

---

[18] Compare with Chapter Five.

cific powers and intensify them greatly. Stones tumbled into a round form, called hand stones, are most suitable. They don't need to be any larger than the size of a cherry for the applications explained in this chapter in order to move enormous subtle energies. However, to give the effect of a Rainbow Reiki Mandala a special orientation, it is considerably more important to clearly define the exact purpose in the ritual of making the mandala than to find the appropriate type of stone for it. So don't worry if therapy with healing stones isn't exactly one of your areas of knowledge. If you would like to become more informed in this respect, look at the books listed in the Commented Bibliography.

The procedure for building a crystal mandala is basically similar to the creation of a plant pattern. For this reason, I will only describe the respective step in the process explained above when there is some sort of deviation from it.

***Step 1:*** Proceed as under Step 1 in the instructions for building plant patterns.

***Step 2:*** Choose at least three stones for the pattern. Hold each of them in your hand for a moment. Greet it, explain what you plan to do with it, and ask if it wants to participate. If you receive a sign of rejection, respect it. The mineral beings usually enjoy being in a mandala and moving energies. But sometimes they don't. Maybe

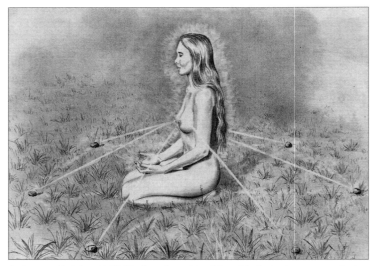

*Sitting in a Rainbow Reiki Healing-Stone Mandala is like being in an energy bath*

they need peace and quiet, purification, some sunlight, or want to first get to know you better and spend some time close to you before they get more deeply involved. Respect this.

The maximum number of stones you can use for a pattern is theoretically unlimited. However, you should be careful with mandalas made of more than 11 individual stones. Rainbow Reiki patterns will objectively never cause you harm, but their power can be so strong that you walk around as if you were in a trance when close to them. Large patterns of more than 11 stones develop an enormous vibrational field that can have a very intensive effect within a radius of 20 meters or more. Think of your neighbors and possible fellow residents, as well as living areas where you perhaps prefer not to experience a certain effect from a pattern. Then you should build a smaller one.

I usually use from a minimum of three to a maximum of nine stones in my work. This is more than enough for most tasks. Various types of stones can be combined very well, but I wouldn't bring together more than four different types in one mandala. The variety of vibrational qualities may otherwise be rather confusing for you if you aren't used to dealing with strong subtle energies on an advanced level.

*Step 3*: Go to the place where you would like to lay out the Rainbow Reiki Mandala. Be sure that you are undisturbed there, and attune yourself to it for a few minutes. At the same time, give yourself Reiki on your heart and forehead chakra. Then spread out all the stones next to you, give them Reiki for a moment, and then feel your way into the vibrations that they are sending out. Think about your plans, then ask the powers of light and love for guidance and carefully pick up all the pieces. Hold them in both hands in front of your heart, give them Reiki and look at them as if they were a person you love. While doing so, sing the mantra "Hey loa, key loa..." nine times. Then hold the stones up to the heavens, look at them with a loving gaze, and also sing the mantra nine times here and give them Reiki. Pause for a moment and perceive the strong, clear power now emanating from the consecrated pieces. Start to sing the song again and continue until the ritual is finished. One after the other, carefully put each object onto the spot where you want to create the mandala. Put down one after the other so that a clear, balanced geometry is created. This is important because of the crystalline structure of the stones, which is very different from that of plants. For example, when you work with three stones, lay out an even-sided triangle. If there are four, lay out a square, and so forth. There are deviations from this principle only in mandalas that are laid out for the direct healing of energy centers (chakras). You will find more information about this in the next section.

When you have laid down everything, wait for a moment, put both your hands on the area of your heart, and thank the powers of light and love. Feel the power of the Rainbow Reiki Mandala, which is now fully capable of functioning. Now it is working and ready to do its job.

**Step 4:** Proceed as under Step 4 in the instructions for building plant patterns.

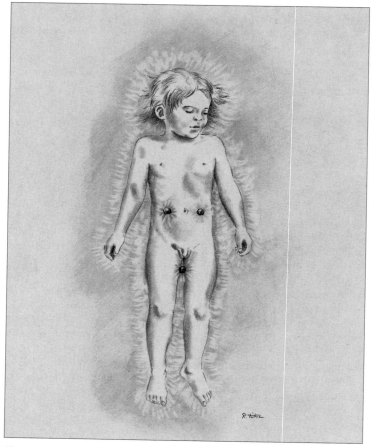

*The Rainbow Reiki Crystal Mandala for natural grounding*

# The Four Main
# Chakra Healing Mandalas

There are four special patterns for purifying, stabilizing, and charging the human energy body. These can be laid out according to the same principle as described above, but with specially chosen stones and a geometry suitable for this respective purpose.

## The Crystal Healing Mandala for Grounding

With this pattern, the energetic structures of the first two chakras in particular are normalized and, when this has taken place, the development of their individual functions, as well as their mutual cooperation, is promoted. It can also be generally used for the stimulation of this energy center in order to prevent imbalances and foster the willingness for further development. If these two chakras function well, a person has the power, endurance, and emotional motivation to make something out of his life. He can better assert himself, accept his body, create playful encounters with others, and enjoy his life in a sensual way. The upper chakras depend on the lower ones for their supply of energy and can only improve their ability to work to the extent that their power is made available to them from below. This is also a reason for the saying: "A happy body is the foundation of spiritual development."

In contrast to the other methods of activating the lower chakras, this healing crystal pattern has the advantage of automatically promoting a natural integration of the increased power into the rest of the energy system by providing controlling information for cross-linking the forces in the body. This prevents one-sided growth.

Despite this, to be on the safe side you should be sure that you don't work with this pattern more often than twice a week with a maximum of 15 minutes at a time. After each session, the soles of the feet should be given Reiki for a few minutes. Hara breathing is also recommended. When you have gathered more experience with this type of energy work, you will be able to judge for yourself what can be tolerated at which point in time and what could bring too much healing at once.

For this pattern, use three tumbled crystal quartz stones in the maximum size of a cherry or a walnut. Activate the crystals as described above. As shown in the illustration on the adjacent page, calmly, consciously, and lovingly lay them on your body or your

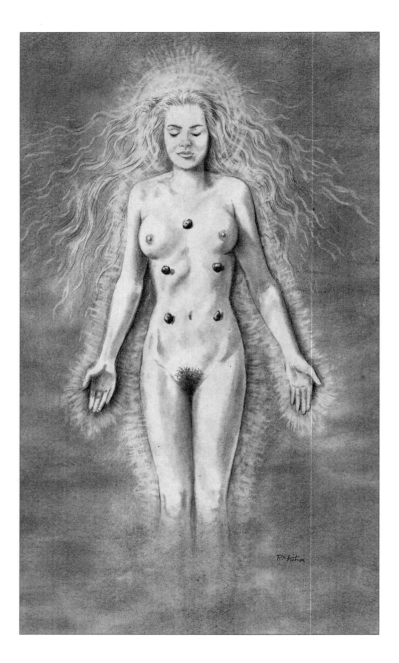

*Rainbow Reiki crystal mandala for developing the ability to have relationships*

exercise partner's body one after the other at a distance of one small handbreadth to the right and left of the navel and about one handbreadth below the crotch.

## The Crystal Healing Mandala
## for Strengthening the Ability to Have Relationships

With this pattern, the 3rd and 4th chakras are purified, stabilized, and strongly charged. This is a precondition for working through fears, creating stronger self-respect, and developing a feeling for the self, as well as supporting the ability to have relationships with others; for love, empathy, tolerance, and being capable of forgiveness.

Use five tumbled rose quartz stones for this pattern in the approximate size of a cherry or walnut. Activate them as described above and lay them out as shown in the adjacent illustration: on a. the heart chakra, b. and c. vertically below the nipples on the level of the solar plexus, and d. and e. to the left and right of the navel, each about one handbreadth from it.

At first, this Rainbow Reiki Mandala should also not be used for more than twice a week and 15 minutes at a time. At its conclusion, again give Reiki to the soles of the feet and have the person receiving treatment breathe into the hara.

## The Crystal Healing Mandala
## for Strengthening Spirituality

With this pattern, the 5th and 6th chakras can be cleared, stabilized, and developed. This results in a growth of self-expression, creativity, intuition, and the certainty of doing the respective right thing for all those involved. The powers of subtle perception are expanded and refined. It is also well-suited for all difficulties that result from too much inner chaos. If a person simply doesn't know how he should plan his life for the long-term and can't find his own path although he generally likes being in this world and participating in its activities, this mandala can help him. It is also recommended for people who want to develop their artistic abilities. Remember to support the harmonious effects of this pattern through complementary work on the lower four energy centers. You know the simple methods from your First Degree course and there are enough advanced ones in this and other books of mine.

All four main Rainbow Reiki Crystal Healing Mandalas strengthen not only the respective chakras, but also provide controlling information

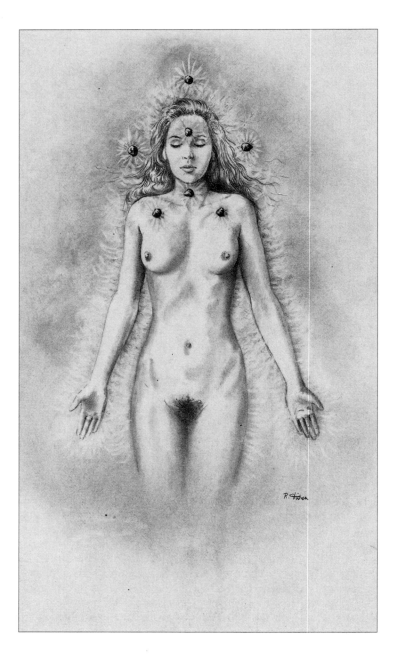

*The Rainbow Reiki Crystal Mandala for supporting spiritual consciousness*

for the newly activated energies. Despite this, they still can't take on everything alone. This would also contradict the spiritual principle of responsibility for oneself. The person who has been given treatment should always also contribute to a more balanced functioning of his major chakras by not living in a one-sided manner.[19] For this pattern, use seven amethysts in the size of about a cherry to a maximum size of a walnut. Activate them as described above and lay them, as shown in the adjacent illustration, a. one handbreadth above the top of the head, b. and c. respectively one handbreadth next to each ear, d. on the throat chakra, e. on the 6th chakra, and f. and g. respectively to the left and right in the hollow directly below the collarbone.

As in the other patterns, this Rainbow Reiki Mandala should not be used more than twice a week for 15 minutes at a time at the start. At its conclusion, once again give Reiki to the soles of the feet for a time and have the person being treated breathe into the hara.

## The Rainbow Reiki Crystal Healing Mandala for Strengthening the Entire Energy System

This pattern is a unique possibility for finely tuning all components of the subtle energy system and strengthening them in relation to each other. After such a session, the aura is frequently five to six times as large and strong as before. It reduces stress and promotes inner harmony. Yet, this mandala is not a substitute for the other three. It cannot penetrate as deeply into the individual energy centers as they can, being responsible instead for their cooperation and the attunement of the aura fields.

For this purpose, use three rose quartz stones, three amethysts, and three crystal quartz stones, making a total of nine stones with the same size, as in the previously described patterns. Activate them as described above. As in the picture on the adjacent page, lay them out as follows: a. one handbreadth above the top of the head (amethyst), b. on the 6th chakra (amethyst), c. on the heart center (amethyst), d. and e. respectively one handbreadth next to the shoulders (rose quartz), f. on the heart chakra (rose quartz), g. and h. respectively on handbreadth next to the pelvis (crystal quartz), and i. (crystal quartz) about one handbreadth below the feet in the middle between them.

At first, don't use this pattern more than once a week for about 15 minutes. At its conclusion, once again give Reiki to the soles of the feet for some time and have the person treated breathe into the hara.

---

[19] I have published an abundance of material on this topic in many other publications and would like to use the space in this book for something new.

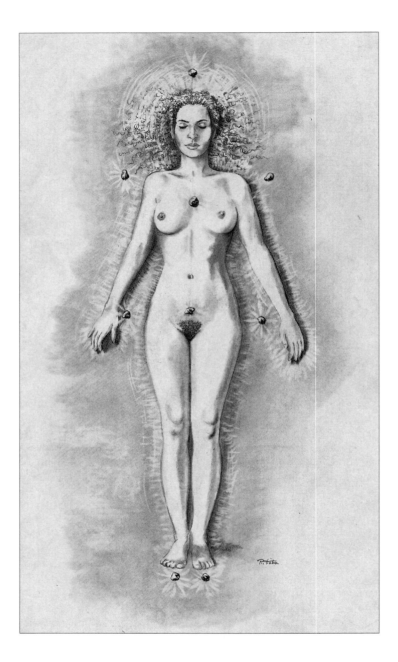

*Rainbow Reiki Crystal Mandala for strengthening the entire energy syystem*

52

The effects of all four patterns are very extensive and can best be understood if you gather experience with them and write it down on a regular basis. Work with the main Rainbow Reiki Crystal Healing Mandalas for yourself and others. When you do this, do something like give a Reiki session or take a fantasy journey at the same time. You will be amazed at what begins to move as a result.

# Examples for Practical Application of Rainbow Reiki Mandalas[20]

There are many possibilities for working with the Rainbow Reiki mandala. Here are some of them:

a. Sit or stand in or next to a pattern, depending on how large it is and how it is constructed. Attune yourself to it by looking at it and widely opening yourself to its beneficial vibrations. Request healing, protection, knowledge, and guidance. Now inhale the energy streaming from the Rainbow Reiki Mandala in calm, deep breaths. Pause each time you inhale and feel how the harmonious energy spreads more and more within you.

b. Establish contact—as described under a.—with the mandala. Use your hands to slowly and consciously draw in the energy emanating from the pattern, about 10 to 20 centimeters above it, for example. Do this as if you were taking water from a well. Bring the light-filled power into your chakras with your hands. Feel your way into the liberating, harmonizing effect each time for a while.

c. Sit or lay down close to the pattern. Establish contact—as described under a.—with the aura emanating from the mandala. Be passive and let the healing power work with you without becoming active yourself.

d. Approach a Rainbow Reiki Mandala and establish contact with it as described under a. Let yourself be intuitively guided by the vibrations of the pattern to dance steps, body positions, and songs. This is also a very effective exercise for the development of your subtle perception.

e. In a correspondingly large Rainbow Reiki Crystal Mandala, give a Reiki session, a massage, or something similar.

f. Make love with your partner within a healing pattern, such as one made of carnelian, rhodochrosite, and fire opals. The two of you will never forget this experience! Before you come together, each of you should individually become attuned within the mandala to

---

[20]The following suggestions do not apply to the previously described four special mandalas!

its vibrations for about 5 to 10 minutes. Then sit facing each other for about 5 to 10 minutes, hold hands, and look into each other's eye so that you enter into a mutual vibration. Then do whatever the two of you find enjoyable.

g. If you have a client with grounding problems, lay out a corresponding grounding mandala around his feet. He should leave his feet close to the pattern for about 15 to 20 minutes. Also give the usual Reiki treatments during this time. It is naturally possible and useful to do this before or afterwards as well.

h. Special Rainbow Reiki Mandalas can be laid out in order to promote a deep, restful sleep, give fearful children a sense of security, impregnate a place with powerful spiritual vibrations in order to purify it of old, disharmonious patterns or prepare it to be a protected area in which energy work and meditation function particularly well.

i. Healing stones of all types, jewelry, water, food, or massage oils can be positively charged and purified in the vicinity of a Rainbow Reiki Mandala or within it. Three to four hours of charging time are usually adequate. However, a longer period of time doesn't hurt but increases the effect within the limitations of the materials.

j. Lay out a Rainbow Reiki Mandala on imbalanced Earth-ray fields in order to create and maintain a life-promoting flow of Earth energies.

k. Take three tumbled crystal quartz stones about as large as a cherry, three rose quartz stones, and three amethysts of the same type in a small medicine bag on trips. You will then always be equipped for all situations and can use a Rainbow Reiki mandala to create a harmonious vibration in your hotel room and a little power place for meditation, regeneration, and relaxation wherever you want, for example, or do healing energy work for yourself and others. Even in a high-rise building, you can easily reach the forces of nature in this way.

# CHAPTER FOUR

# Rainbow Reiki and Work With Friends from Subtle Dimensions

An important area of Rainbow Reiki is the contact, exchange, and meaningful human work, equally beneficial to all involved, with beings that live in the subtle planes of our universe. These beings have been known everywhere in the world among those with esoteric interests since the beginning of human existence. They have been given many names, such as: fairies, angels, nature spirits, power animals, devas, or elves. They have been given a great spectrum of esteem, ranging from uncritical worship and veneration to complete rejection, fear, and "demonization." At the same time, they are neither gods nor devils. In some respects, they are different from human beings—however, in others they have some things in common with us.

My own experiences with subtle beings of all types began during early childhood. Fascinated by what I was permitted to experience, I have theoretically and practically encountered all the sources of this topic to which I have had access time and again since then. After I received the Second Reiki Degree, a new, wonderful world, which I had not believed possible despite my previous knowledge, opened up for me in this respect. I soon discovered a series of expansions of certain Second Degree techniques that made it possible for me to establish contact and communicate with a great variety of inhabitants of other dimensions in a way that is quick, simple, and without the unavoidable, extensive safety measures otherwise required for journeys into other planes of existence. The experiences gathered in the previous years were of help to me since establishing contact, feeling good about it, making oneself understood, and being understood don't necessarily go hand in hand. There are also specific rules of behavior for dealing with beings of the subtle worlds, and it is useful and often absolutely necessary to adhere to them in order to have a meaningful effect.

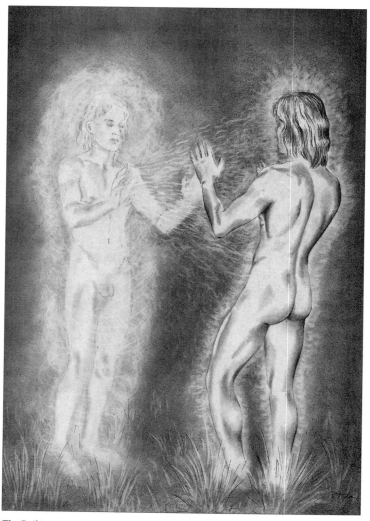

*The Reiki contact with your Higher Self helps you realize your plan in life*

# Subtle Beings Aren't "Substitute Gods"

The beings that I write about here are not God and also don't want to be a substitute for God. They are somewhat ahead of many people in this respect. They are children of the one God, the Creator of everything that is, just as we are. Among them are specialists with a great variety of knowledge, abilities, preferences, aversions, and needs. As outstanding as we may often view their possibilities to be, we human beings have some capabilities that are completely obvious to us, but appear incomprehensible and enormous from their perspective. When we know this, we can work together in an egalitarian manner with the inhabitants of other planes and learn from each other without forgetting that each of us has had a good reason for choosing an incarnation and therefore an emphasis of experience on a certain level of existence for a specific amount of time. The many different levels of existence, and all those who live on them, are equally valuable to the Creation in the overall context. As soon as hierarchic thinking in one direction or the other develops, meaning an attitude of "being better or worse than this being" in the contacts with the subtle forces, an end is put to any type of meaningful cooperation from the spiritual perspective.

Before we take a closer look at our subtle friends, who I also like to call the inhabitants of other dimensions, in a practical way, I want to tell you a bit more about the theoretical background of the methods necessary for this purpose so that you know exactly what this is about and on which foundation this very special form of Rainbow Reiki energy work is constructed.

## Theoretical Foundations for Contacts and Work with Subtle Beings

Our universe consists of many different planes of existence, separated from each other in a certain respect by energetic structures. What we human beings normally experience in our everyday life is just one of these areas of being. There are comprehensive natural laws that are valid in every dimension such as that love causes liveliness to occur. Others only apply to certain areas, such as the law ruling the course of time or the existence of space, meaning the separation of the individual parts of the Creation by differences in time and space. Some rules are also exclusively effective in one area alone. There is life on practically all levels of the universe, even if it sometimes takes on extremely exotic forms from the human perspective. At the same time, every form of life is fundamentally adapted to the energetic plane of existence in which it is born and currently lives. It spends its everyday life there, gathers the lion's share of its experiences, particularly in the formative early childhood, and it is not truly permitted to permanently flee from the basic laws of its homeland before its death. However, it is possible under certain conditions for it to temporarily explore other areas of the Creation, become active there, and maintain contact with the beings that live there. This is a result of the structure of life itself, which is ultimately unlimited and unlimitable. The connection to a plane for a certain amount of time from birth there (awakening of the existential consciousness for this dimension) until death there (shifting of the existential consciousness from the previous plane of development to another) is basically just a strong emphasis on certain mechanisms of perception and action, as well as a (desired) limitation of a being's ability of consciousness. Through this voluntarily made choice of the existential emphasis of consciousness (everyday life), made before incarnation in a certain area of the Creation, essentially more intensive and, above all, truly new experiences are possible. These are more necessary for the development of the personality and ultimately for the entire Creation than if all planes would be constantly accessible for the consciousness of a being. However, when an individual being comprehends its freedom through liberating personal development, learning to use it in a loving and responsible manner, it is capable of sharing advice and helping not only with other inhabitants of its own level of existence (horizontal cross-linking of life), but also deliberately establishing contact with other planes and the creatures living there, working together with them for their mutual benefit (vertical cross-linking of life). In ancient times this vertical cross-linking was quite common, respected, and carried out systematically. Today, it is still customary among the native peoples, the so-called primitive races. In the Western industrial nations, an interest in this has started to develop once again. The renaissance of shamanism[21], for example, is a sign of this development.

# The Iceberg Principle:
# Your Everyday Life Happens at the Focus
# of Your Consciousness Work

The "iceberg principle" is what I call an important concept that perhaps permits the multidimensional concept of life and the possibilities of vertical cross-linking with subtle beings to become more comprehensible. You are certain to know that only a small part of the iceberg juts out of the water and is visible, while a considerably larger portion rests beneath the surface of the water. The multidimensional structures of living beings can also be understood in a similar manner. Take a tree as an example. What you normally see, hear, or feel of it is just one part of its entire existence, namely what is directly perceptible on our level of existence and subject to its laws. The part of it that is directly tangible on this level usually has just a minor power of consciousness[22] so that we humans perceive it to be less developed than an animal or person. The other parts of the tree being are only revealed to those who have learned to deal with their subtle senses and possibilities of action in an expanded manner. As soon as you are in the position of gathering information on more than one level of existence, you will be able to convince yourself that trees, in parts of their being that exist in other dimensions, also have a more highly developed consciousness and considerably more extensive possibilities than may be presumed from their appearance in this world. The native peoples of America call the abilities and personality parts of plants, animals, minerals, and elements concealed in the subtle planes "medicine power" and have included it in their lives for thousands of years. In Nordic mythology, this principle is expressed by the archetypal tree Yggdrasil, in whose branches the various worlds of the gods, human beings, elves, dwarfs, and giants exist. In Eastern esoterics, the Cabalistic Tree of Life describes the same contents with different terms.

## Subtle Helper Powers
## The Invisible Friends

On some levels, but not only there, beings who would like to take part in work on the cross-linking and development of life in the greater context prefer to incarnate because they want to learn something and further develop themselves in this respect. They have a series of abilities that are very useful and far-reaching for this purpose. One of the basic laws that these "folks" must learn, which gives them a considerable portion of their wonderful powers at the same time, is: "Only become active for others when you are requested to do so!" Only when the freedom of a being in relation to the shaping of its own life is guaranteed can it harmoniously fit into

---

[21] Also compare with the Appendix on Reiki and the contact with the healing powers of nature by Greta-Bahya Hessel-Lübeck.
[22] If it has much consciousness in it on this level, it will become a great place of power, a holy or healing tree.

the universal order and meaningfully participate in the Creation's evolution.

Among other things, these helper forces build lines of communication between the various levels of the Creation, watch over the power places as "protectors of the place," and make sure that the life-preserving streams of energy can circulate freely between all levels and reach all beings that are prepared with respect to their state of development[23] to receive the respective power qualities and therefore desire the contact. Pan, Cernunnos, plant devas, protectors of the animals, and guardian angels are names that some of these friendly creatures have received in our world. Don't confuse what these beings are and what they actually do with what certain circles propagate about them in order to secure political, economic, and pseudo-spiritual monopolies for themselves. Form your own opinion by gathering experiences with them and evaluating them without prejudice.

# Human Beings Also Have Subtle Portions with Immense Hidden Powers

Human beings also have subtle portions in other dimensions with latently existing, extensive possibilities. However, since the consciousness of most people is concentrated in this level of existence, these talents can't be used in a controlled way without practice and an expanded consciousness. Only in the course of genuine spiritual process of development (in which increasingly larger portions of one's own being are lovingly integrated into consciousness), and by accepting responsibility for one's own life as the precondition for more extensive participation in the evolution of the comprehensive life structures (Creation), do the hidden subtle powers become gradually accessible. Then they soon become a quite naturally applied means of shaping one's life. A more or less *short-term* opportunity for using limited subtle abilities is often granted by the subtle

---

[23] Please don't interpret reference to a certain state of development in the hierarchic sense. Instead, consider every being as an equally important and meaningful level of development, but each individual being can only be open for very specific things in a thematic sense. If you are "spiritually developed," this doesn't mean that you leave others behind who are less "wise," but that you personally learn to deal with the your changing themes of experience and experiences in a very effective way. Even spiritually developed beings make mistakes and can only receive and use new abilities and possibilities when they—as applies to all others as well—give up something in the same proportion. Even for "developed" beings, incarnations don't take place on a ladder because they are "well-behaved," but so that new experiences become possible, meaningfully complementing those gathered beforehand.

helper forces as a touchstone for a person's consciousness of responsibility, as an incentive and challenge for completely new experiences, as help in an emergency situation, or as a catalyst for social transformation. According to the way in which the expanded abilities are approached as an available potential, they stagnate, regress, or continue to be developed in the person who has received them or in the society in general, if this is holistically meaningful for something or someone. As a result, a person provided with subtle powers isn't necessarily competent in the spiritual sense as a teacher or holistic healer. There can be many reasons for his exotic abilities. Taking these facts into consideration, think about the consequences for involvement with the Usui System of Reiki/Rainbow Reiki and its permanence as a tradition. It may depend on us and our attitude whether Reiki remains available for everyone in the long term, if even children will once again come into the world with this ability or if it will again go underground and can only be used by very few people with great efforts on their part.

Becoming aware of the deep solidarity with all life in our world and making the effort to take into account this cross-linking, maintaining it, and helping develop it is a great step. An even greater step is understanding that our level of existence is just one part of the universe with its living souls, that every being exists in all dimensions, and that in this respect the maintenance and intensification of the cooperation of each one with all others is not only important for the development of one's own personality, but also represents a significant contribution to the evolution of the entire Creation.

Rainbow Reiki methods offer comparably simple, and yet extremely effective and expandable ways of increasing the possibilities of perception and activity, up into other levels of existence. However, in order for these journeys to bring meaningful results, it is important to know the best way in which to approach the ensuing subtle perceptions and what should be heeded in contacts with beings whose home lies in other areas of the Creation and whose life is determined in part by laws other than our own.

# Rules of Behavior for Involvement with Subtle Beings

First and most important, be clear about the fact that subtle beings are not God or substitutes for God. They are *not* all-knowing, omnipotent, and perfect. They can only do certain things much better than we humans—and other things they do much worse. For example, a power animal can be a very good adviser and helper in order to cure psychosomatic afflictions, harmonize relationship problems, or more effectively perform and understand certain types of energy work. On the other hand, it would be hopelessly overtaxed with doing the dishes, repairing the car, or mowing the lawn and admires these abilities in human beings.

Always treat your partners with courtesy and respect, but never with subservience. Honor their wishes and advice, but never misunderstand them to be commands. *Always* keep the responsibility for your life plan in your own hands! Your subtle friends may put you to the test in order to determine whether you are already suited for deeper knowledge, more intensive possibilities of energetic action, or certain important projects. If you uncritically hand over the responsibility for your life to them or if you do what they apparently want you to do without stopping to think whether this will promote the *consciousness*, *ability to love*, and *personal responsibility* of all participants, they will withdraw somewhat from you and limit their work with you to a degree safe for all sides until your development has grown accordingly and you can be active to a greater extent without creating shambles. The same happens when they impart something to you that you don't use in a practical sense in the following period of time, and despite this, still want to have more knowledge or possibilities from the next contact. Furthermore, the subtle teachers refuse to impart knowledge that just will be for the sake of sensation or satisfaction of other superficial needs on the part of the person requesting it. Also, only ask for things that you really need and want to use. Always give some thought in advance to whether you can actually master the corresponding task only through energy work. If there are conventional ways of doing it, use these first!

## Finding the Right Partner for a Certain Purpose

Subtle beings each have very special, unique talents. For this reason, when selecting your "workmate" for a project, be sure that it is actually suited for it. I will give an exact explanation of how to make such a choice later. To be on the safe side, before beginning the actual work ask whether it even wants to do it and considers itself suitable for the task.

Successful Communication with Beings of the Subtle Planes Means the Ability to Read Between the Lines.

The communication with beings of the subtle planes seldom takes place as directly as that of the customary level between human beings. You can assume that the truly important messages are expressed between the lines. Learn to understand their behavior, the experiences they share with you, and the perceptions they make possible for you as metaphors for what they want to tell you. Only in very few cases will a subtle adviser say to you: "Do this, don't do that!"[24] You will usually receive messages that you must decode through hard, but very instructive detailed work. Or the subtle teachers will ask you questions, which they particularly like to do. I sometimes think it's practically a type of sport for them. The constant questioning can be a bother, but it is ultimately a wonderful way of learning to contemplate something and feel what's going on inside yourself in an effective, guided manner. In addition, it also trains your own ability to learn in the spiritual sense.

Some other special qualities that many subtle beings have represent a source of great misunderstanding:
a. They take you literally and believe that you already know why you do or don't want to have something. As long as this doesn't contradict the cosmic order and you give them a suitable present in return or they are the teachers personally responsible for you and have had much experience with people and their special character traits, they will make an effort to fulfill your request.
b. They only come when they are called.
c. They only disappear when you have officially taken leave of them or they become bored.

**On a.**
How can something like this cause difficulties, you want to know?!
Unfortunately, many people don't give intensive thought to whether what they want from the forces, even just as they expresss it, is suitable for making them happy.

**On b.**
It could be that nothing happens when something is supposed to happen because simply no one has made an official request to the

---

[24] There is an entire series of cases in which people channel supposed subtle beings that do nothing but give instructions from morning to night. However, closer investigation has determined that such "teachers" tend to be suppressed parts of the channel's personality with extensive, incompatible claims to power. A person who wants to make other people into marionettes is not suited as a teacher for spiritual development—no matter what he calls himself and how bombastically he performs. A strong aura doesn't necessarily mean that a person has good intentions and a mature personality. Hitler also had charisma and persuasive powers and was able to lead many people to their ruin because they delegated their responsibility to him and took action without seriously becoming conscious of the resulting consequences.

subtle worlds and taken into consideration a fair exchange (exchange = offering; see explanation on this further down!). People are then quick to say: "This doesn't even work!"

## On c.

Things constantly happen that weren't even desired because the forces that have been summoned were given abundant gifts, but no one told them exactly what they should do. Instead of sitting around doing nothing, they then react to every concentrated, strongly emotional thought and try to become active, with the above-mentioned limitations, according to these "instructions." If they are not expressly sent away, they also like to stay (in as far as they have nothing more important to do) and develop activities until they think that they have done their part for the offering given to them. In case someone forgot to tell them or they are not clearly told that their work is finished for the moment and they are officially dismissed, they stay and understand every thought strongly connected with intensive emotions in the area of the place to which they have been called to be instructions for action. And as long as these "orders" are not in direct contradiction to the cosmic order on principle, they like to put them into practice...

   Last but not least, you should never establish contact with the beings of the subtle planes when you are extremely agitated emotionally or strongly moved by the theme that is to be worked on, when you are very tired, or extremely stressed[25]. You should also never try to work with the spirits in order to harm someone or create a profit for yourself without a service in return. Under these specified conditions, there is a great probability that you won't understand the subtle messages from the other dimensions or not understand them correctly, act in a thoughtless manner and deal with the subtle beings (which are quite vulnerable in a certain sense) in a way that is too coarse, or attempt to put yourself in opposition to the universal order. This would not only endanger the implementation of your current plan, but possibly also make your work with the spirits more difficult for a long time to come and perhaps also set things in motion that you would *very* much regret afterwards. You should therefore always heed to these points, which will then eliminate the most frequent and serious causes of "interdimensional relationship problems."

---

[25]Exceptions to the points mentioned in this sentence are your Higher Self and your Inner Child, as well as such beings as a guardian angel or power animal you have already consciously worked with for a longer period of time and is familiar with your special qualities.

## The Offering—A Frequently Completely Misunderstood Principle of Fair Exchange According to the Laws of Divine Order

When you receive something important for you, you should give something that is just as valuable to your exchange partner in the sense of the cosmic order—otherwise, "bad karma" is created. This thought is the basis for offerings to subtle beings. When you give something that you urgently need yourself to survive, to be healthy, or to have experiences that are important for you, it is an act of self-punishment but not at all in keeping with the natural laws. Plants give oxygen to human beings and animals. If they would keep it, this highly reactive element would burn and poison them. For plants, oxygen is a dangerous waste product of their metabolism. For us, it is the elixir of life—without it we would have to die within minutes. The carbon dioxide that we exhale serves plants as an important nutrient. They live from it. We would suffocate if we kept it for ourselves. If human beings would give off oxygen and plants release carbon dioxide, the healthy cycle of life-maintaining give-and-take would be interrupted and all those participating in it would suffer a miserable end. The laws of nature apply to energy work and the work with subtle beings. When we respect them, our actions will always have a beneficial effect for all involved in the sense of the cosmic order, meaning "good karma."

In return for their services in healing, for example, shamans give the spirits ritually consecrated tobacco, flour, milk, honey, or fragrant essences. On the subtle plane, the burning of certain objects or substances in a specific ritual process also releases qualities that the beings living there find very pleasant and can put to good use for themselves.

The release of strong feelings under circumstances harmonizing with the respective purpose can also be a suitable return service. This is the basis of many tantric rituals. Sometimes the spirits would like for a person who works with them to do something for them that is important in our world or their world, but they alone can't manage it or have a difficult time doing so. They never ask for an offering that reduces the ability to love, the consciousness, or the personal responsibility of the person involved! Quite to the contrary: an offering in the sense of the cosmic order always detoxifies the giver in the material, energetic, emotional, or psychological sense. Things that are obstructing him are taken away and new free space, more strength, and health are created for him, just like the "oxygen offering" of a plant keeps it healthy and permits its metabolism to function.

For the greatest variety of reasons, people naturally hang onto precisely the energies, material things, ways of behaving, and feel-

65

ings that do lasting damage to themselves and perhaps even their environment, preventing personal holistic growth. In such a case, the offering that a subtle being proposes may appear to be cruel, painful, or senseless.

Perhaps it is also one of the tests mentioned above and isn't even desirable for you to give what has been described. Instead, you are meant to politely but definitely refuse the demand and independently choose to give something more suitable. You can discover this by reflection, feeling what's going on inside yourself, and perhaps talking to friends and doing oracle work. No matter what the end result is: this path will make you stronger and more capable of happiness. Plus—it's fun and can be very exciting.

## Reiki as an Offering

"Reikians" can do something good for their subtle friends at any time: namely, provide them with Reiki! This may sound like carrying coals to Newcastle, but don't assume that the inhabitants of others planes of existence also master every form of energy work that some humans can do. This may be the case, and it may not. In addition: even if some spirits can also work with Reiki, wouldn't you also like to receive a Reiki treatment from others once in a while and simple enjoy it, without having to do anything yourself? They feel the same way. Furthermore, there are projects that need many beings working on them so that they can succeed. How Reiki can be given to subtle beings as a return service in accordance with the First or Second Degree will be described in more detail in the practice section of this chapter. However, it is important not to exclude the opportunity of sacrificing something that burdens you when you would be better off giving it as an offering. You can naturally also give Reiki along with it in any case. Give thought time and again to the most suitable offering in each respective case. And don't believe you have nothing that you shouldn't get rid of. There's always something; you do exhale once in a while, don't you?

# Addressing Subtle Beings
# in an Appropriate Manner

There is a traditional way of addressing the spirits or a Higher Self that you can always use at the beginning when you establish contact with them. This is not a matter of learning something word-for-word by heart, but consciously duplicating the meaning. It's best for you to find your own words after you have felt your way into the following text.

> *I come to you as an unhealthy person and request healing. I come to you as an ignorant person and ask for teaching. I come to you as a helpless person and ask for support and protection. I come to you as a powerless person and ask for power in order to better serve. In return for your services, I offer you (name offering quality—Reiki, for example).*

For ending the contact, the following text can be used.

> *I thank you for your cooperation and support. The time of our contact is over for now. I ask that you come to me again when I call you (alternative: that I can again come to you). Now return to your home. May light, love, and the blessing of the creative power be with you!*

You should basically use these forms of address as an opening and closing in all contacts with Higher Selves, power animals, angels, or other subtle friends. In the following exercises, I will assume that you remember to do this every time.

# Contact Training with Angels, Medicine Animals, and Other Exotic Friends

In this section, I have compiled a complete training program for contact and effective work with subtle beings. Do yourself a favor and assume that you need it! I can well understand that you are very much itching to start further down, but that probably wouldn't work out quite right at this point. You have the best prospects for success if you first learn the ABCs before starting to write a novel. Believe me, I'm speaking from my own experience. I didn't exactly inherit an attitude of patience either...

## Input
**Possibilities of perception/ senses**

## Output
**Possibilities of expression and manipulation**

---

# Higher Self

Level of relative unity of time and space. Tasks: Supervision of life plan/ advice for life in holistic sense/ function of spiritual healer/ inner healer in holistic sense

Direct perception of all levels of existence

"Coincidences," oracle determined by coincidence

# Middle Self

Level of analysis/material world Task area: Solution of problems in "here and now". Rational understanding and manipulation of the world. Setting goals for the future and understanding the past. Constructive realization of emotional energies. Creation of unconscious patterns of thinking and acting to facilitate shaping of life.

All "normal senses" like sight, hearing, smell, touch, kinesthetic sense

Language, conscious physical expression that is created by physical expression through unconscious pattern of thinking and acting

# Inner Child

Level of synthesis/magic/ mysticism Task area: Acquiring power for contact with Creation on material level and being willing to use it to shape your life. Storing memories/ letting feelings flow as the necessary synthetic complement to the judgment of the analytic mind. Inner healer and teacher in the magical-shamanic sense.

The so-called subtle energetic senses: telepathy, emotional telepathy, clairvoyance and clairsentience, precognition, the use of the pendulum, retrocognition, the ability to see areas, and many other types of energy perception.

Magical-energetic manipulations like psychokinesis, sympathetic magic, transmission of psychologically effective energies. Teleportation, levitation, materialization, etc. Physical expression of emotional energies.

*"Trust me, I know what I'm doing...!"*
Freely quoted according to "Sledge Hammer"

An important precondition for every type of energy work is the best possible integration of a person's Inner Child into his overall personality. The term "Inner Child" comes from the HUNA teaching, an old spiritual tradition widespread in the Pacific region that has a great many congruences with the traditions upon which Dr. Usui developed his method of natural healing with Reiki. There is a series of indications that the Reiki method was even developed a long, long time ago in this region. But that's another story...

Back to the Inner Child: It's the part of a person that contains and controls his memory, feelings and instincts, vitality, and abilities of subtle perception and energy work. The Inner Child doesn't have much use for logic, but it likes to play, is enormously creative, and has excellent abilities of perceiving comprehensive correlations and patterns. It loves metaphors, sensual pleasures, and is therefore closely connected with the body and the physical nature in general. In the following exercise, using the Reiki Two method you can establish contact with your Inner Child and give it Reiki directly. If you carry out this exercise on a regular basis at intervals that aren't too long, your Inner Child will be connected more and more with your overall personality and make itself noticeable in your consciousness in many ways. Be sure to respect its perspective of the world, which is completely different from your conscious, rational portion, the Middle Self. Permit yourself to dream and play more, to pay more attention to your body and its needs, and to feel and express more emotions. Then you will perhaps get to know a previously unimagined degree of vitality, creativity, and joy in life.

If you want to make contact with subtle beings, you should build up the contact to your Inner Child beforehand over a longer period of time, ask it for help in every plan in this direction, and keep the connection with it until you have ended the corresponding work with the subtle being. Then say goodbye to it and thank it for its support. In a number of respects, your Inner Child can be a great help to you in working with the inhabitants of other planes of existence.

One rule applies to all Reiki distance contacts: you should only work consciously with them. This means that you should only establish a distance contact when your entire attention can be with the connection—otherwise, don't do it! When the time in which you want to have your attention free for the contact is over, end it carefully and consciously, as taught in your Second Degree basic course. It is an error to believe that a constant distance contact with your Higher Self, for example, is important and meaningful. *En-*

*ergy work and personal development only occur to the degree that your attention is with what you are doing.* If you develop your self quickly and securely and would like to learn to deal with higher forms of energy work, as described in this book, become accustomed to doing everything in this regard in a controlled and conscious manner. Consumer-thinking and "a lot helps a lot" have nothing to do with spirituality and esoterics!

You will find one version of the following exercise for the First Degree explained in point 1 b. With the First Degree, you can also do something for an Inner Child, but it takes much longer because you must take a detour in the absence of Second Degree "tools." But don't be sad because of this since you will learn a great deal about your body and its relationship to the Inner Child as a result. In addition, as has already been mentioned before: The path is the ... okay, I don't want to get on your nerves.

### Exercise 1: Strengthening the Connection to Your Inner Child

a. Use the two symbols responsible for the Reiki distance treatment and the corresponding mantras, as well as the form of addressing the "Inner Child of (add first and last name of person to whose Inner Child the contact is to be established)." Turn the palms of your hands away from your body and imagine that there, where they are directed, is the Inner Child. *But don't try to visualize it!* Let it take the initiative and simply wait to see what happens. Use some of the intensification signs and the corresponding mantras in order to provide it with more Reiki.

After every exercise session, which should last three to five minutes once or twice a week and can later also be lengthened as you desire, briefly note your perceptions during the contact in a special book in which you can also write your experiences with Rainbow Reiki energy work in the future. Don't forget the date.

During the contact with your Inner Child, let your attention wander through your entire body and pay attention to any changes in comparison to the state before the contact. Which thoughts are going through your head? Do certain feelings awaken within you or do certain memories or desires suddenly surface within you? All this could be the Inner Child's first attempts to establish contact with you. Don't expect any 3-D pictures and angelic Inner Child figures who proclaim to you some sort of wise sayings, important messages for humanity, or prophecies of the future. Such things aren't very interesting for the Inner Child. Assume that you will need an entire series of sessions until your work with it takes on concrete forms. If it goes more quickly, that's great! Remember to carefully take leave after every distance contact.

b. If you aren't yet initiated into the Second Degree, but are in the First Degree, carry out the exercise in the following manner: lay one hand—it doesn't matter which one since both transmit the same energy because of the initiation into Reiki—with the inner side on your lower belly, just above the pubic bone (2nd chakra) and the other between your legs with the palm of the hand turned towards your crotch (1st chakra). Stay in this position for 10 to 15 minutes and let Reiki be drawn in. As described under a., be sure to watch for changes in your perception and don't expect anything specific, which means that all the more things can happen as a result! Take notes on your experiences afterwards. According to experience, the contact with your Inner Child usually takes longer. It could also be that it immediately makes itself noticeable to you. In any case, leave it the freedom to do so in a form that is pleasant for it and don't demand anything of it.

# Reiki and Your Higher Self

Your Higher Self watches over your life plan and, when your organize your life in a way that deviates from it, tries to show you that what you are doing isn't so good for you and what would be better for you from its point of view. When doing so, it never makes rules but respects the freedom of the Middle Self and the Inner Child in directing one's own life. Its advice can be more frequent, clear, and strong if it is provided with additional energy from the Middle Self, the part of the personalty representing a person's everyday consciousness in the narrower sense. Contacts with your Higher Self on a regular basis have the additional advantage that you can also increasingly integrate this portion with its special abilities (see graphic on pg. 91) and consciously include it in your life. Remember that a Higher Self is on a level of the Creation where time and space are not what they represent in our everyday world. It judges life, morality, and ethics from a vastly different perspective than the Middle Self or even the Inner Child.

Despite all the fantastic possibilities that Higher Selves have, they are not perfect, all-knowing, or omniscient. So don't confuse a Higher Self with God! A Higher Self, a Middle Self, and an Inner Child form the totality of a human being—you, for example! No more and no less. If you put a portion of yourself on a pedestal, a hierarchic structure will develop that impedes the evolution of other parts or even makes it impossible. The Higher Self, Inner Child, and Middle Self are equally important parts with different approaches to life and the world. Every part has its strengths and weaknesses that the other two don't have. So they can learn to complement each other in their cooperation and thereby have a greater effect than as in the sum of the individual parts. The equal cooperation of all three partial personalities is one of the greatest challenges within the scope of genuine spiritual development.

You can also find the concept of the Trinity in practically every religion and spiritual tradition in the world. In Christianity, for example: Father, Son, and Holy Spirit ("Divine Mother" in the original texts that are inaccessible to the public for the most part). In Nordic mythology, it is Odin, Vili, and Ve. In Hinduism, it is Brahma, Vishnu, and Shiva. "As above, so below!" is the old esoteric law, attributed to Hermes Trismegistos, one of the great spiritual teachers of antiquity. As it is for human beings, so it also is, in a greater context, for the divine forces that created and maintain the world and provide for the constant completion of the Creation.

In the distance contacts of the Second Reiki Degree, the special qualities of the existence plane of the Higher Selves—relative lack of time and space—are systematically used in order to be able to send the universal life energy over any desired distance without loss of time or effect, for example. Reiki treatments in the past and future are therefore possible. Unfortunately, there is not enough room for me to go into more detail about these exciting applications here.

If you frequently connect with your Higher Self through the methods described below and send it Reiki indirectly—by the means of the First Degree—or directly, by the means of the Second Degree—the preconditions for better cooperation between all three parts of the personality will be created. This naturally isn't a process that begins today and ends tomorrow! However, you will soon feel many beneficial effects of these types of efforts. Your Higher Self can also serve you well, together with your Inner Child, as a guide and helper in all types of work with other Higher Selves or subtle beings. If you get stuck at some point, give both of them plenty of Reiki and ask for support. If there is a solution for your problem, they will then do their best to help you. At the same time, never forget to be consciously aware of the continued responsibility for how you live your life. Otherwise, you won't really get any further even if you give your Higher Self and your Inner Child Reiki 24 hours a day. They always "just" provide assistance for your Middle Self to help itself. Which isn't all that bad...

## Exercise 2: Strengthening the Connection to Your Higher Self

a. Use the distance treatment symbol, the energy intensification symbol, as well as the corresponding mantras. Clearly direct the Reiki distance contact by using the address form of "Higher Self of (add first and last name of person whose Higher Self you want to contact)." Turn the palms of your hands away from your body and imagine that the Higher Self is at the place where they are directed. But don't try to visualize it in front of your mind's eye! Leave it the initiative and simply wait to see what happens. Use several intensification signs and the respective corresponding manta in order to provide it with more Reiki. Don't forget to take leave from the contact! In no case should you let it constantly continue!

The explanation given in Exercise 1a. also applies to this exercise.

b. If you are initiated into the First Degree, put one hand on your 6th major chakra and the other on your 5th in order to strengthen your connection to your Higher Self. Remain in this position for 10 to 15 minutes and let Reiki be drawn in. At the same time, formulate the wish to come into contact with your Higher Self.[26] As described under 1 a., pay attention to any changes in your perception and don't expect anything in particular—which means all the more that can happen! Afterwards, take notes on your experiences.

According to experience, the contact to your Higher Self usually takes longer with the First Degree. But it's also possible that it quickly makes you aware of its presence here. In any case, permit it the freedom to do this in the form that it finds most suitable and don't make any stipulations.

## Exercise 3a: Creating a Connection with a Power Animal Through Your Higher Self

This exercise only functions satisfactorily when you have been initiated into the Second Degree.

Establish contact with your Higher Self as explained under 2a. Tell it that you would like to get to know a power animal that can help you in the work on a certain problem or generally in the development of your personality at this time. Use further intensification symbols and the corresponding manta in order to provide your Higher Self with more Reiki for this task. Now wait until an animal, no matter what

---

[26] In case you are wondering why I didn't already write this in the exercise for connecting with the Inner Child: This isn't necessary because it basically acts differently than the Higher Self. But it wouldn't hurt at all for you to also ask it to come closer to you.

type, appears in front of your inner eye. When you perceive one, ask whether it would like to work with you. If it acts unwilling or disinterested, ask what you can do so that it supports you. If you still don't receive a positive reaction, respectfully say goodbye to the spirit, no matter how it has acted towards you. This could be a test to see whether you are emotionally stable and mature enough for this type of work. Don't believe that you can deceive a subtle being, it would immediately smell a rat and you would lose the opportunity of getting to know a subtle being more closely for a long time to come.

Ask your Higher Self to mediate a more suitable contact for you. If this doesn't work out either, then respectfully take leave for the time being, give thanks for the help and the experience, and make the connection to search for a power animal later. It is quite possible that you must carry out this exercise for a longer time before you get concrete results. Be patient and take this as a test of your sincerity. Perhaps you can ask an oracle what you could also do in order to create the preconditions for a contact with subtle beings. The Pendulum Table No. 14 in the Appendix is also quite suited for this purpose.

In the general sense, this exercise is suitable for making contact with all types of subtle beings. Don't forget to take leave of a Reiki distance contact every time!

### Exercise 3b: Choosing and Making Contact with a Power Animal by Using the Medicine Cards

Bear and Company in Santa Fe, New Mexico published in 1988 an excellent instrument for work with power animals: the *Medicine Cards, The Discovery of Power Through the Ways of Animals* by Jamie Sams and David Carson. If you want to find a suitable power animal for yourself according to the oracle principle, which means in cooperation with your Higher Self, ask the question: "Which power animal can help me develop my personality?" or "Which power animal can help me solve the problem (add description of problem)?" Then mix the cards and draw one of them while you are thinking of your question. Now you know who can help you.

As an alternative to the *Medicine Cards*, you can also use the Power Animal Pendulum Tables in the Appendix. According to how much experience you have with the pendulum, it may possibly be not quite as effective as the cards, but it also trains further abilities within you. Using the pendulum doesn't function like an oracle through the Higher Self, but through your Inner Child portion.

*If you have been initiated into the First Degree,* you can work together with a power animal by frequently laying on your hands to give Reiki to the corresponding card, some other picture of a representative of this species, or a corresponding stuffed animal for 15 minutes or longer with the intention of sending it to the power animal. This symbolic action can, connected with respectful requests for help, have an effect. For specific reasons, this type of contact functions only with power animals and comparable beings. This technique isn't suitable for Reiki distance treatments of human beings!

The distance contact is often quicker and more versatile. With the tools of the Second Degree, you can establish the contact with the subtle friend in the following manner:

Use the distance treatment sign, the energy intensification sign, as well as the corresponding mantras. Then direct the distance contact through the repeated address form "Higher Self of (add the name of this type of animal)." Turn your hands away from your body with the intention of the power animal being where they are directed. Leave it up to the spirit being whether or not it appears and how it appears in front of your inner eye. Intensify the flow of Reiki energy several times. Otherwise, there's nothing you need to do. If possible, make daily contact to your helper in this way and wait to see what happens. Don't forget to always take leave of every distance contact!

### Exercise 4: Training Your Subtle Perception: Paint a Meditation Picture Together with a Power Animal

This exercise is only suitable for the Second Degree.[27]

Lay out a drawing block and colored pencils. Establish a Reiki distance connection with your Inner Child and your Higher Self. As explained in the last exercise for the Second Degree, establish a distance contact with a power animal. Intensify the flow of the Reiki energy several times. Ask the power animal to draw a meditation picture with your hands. Without giving it much thought, reach for the pencils and let your hands draw a picture. Don't think about how it should be drawn and don't try to control anything! Simply watch as the picture is created. You will sense when it's done. Don't forget to thank your exercise partners and carefully end every Reiki contact that you have established for this exercise.

Before going to sleep every night, focus your attention on the picture that your power animal drew for you for about five minutes. Don't try to analyze it! Just meditate on it. With time, the picture will set into motion a growth process within you and help dissolve blocks. Pay attention to your dreams!

---

[27] There are naturally other methods of reaching a similar result, but not in the Reiki system. Shamanism, wicca, magic, and the like offer a series of tested tools for this purpose. However, these cannot be used "cold." A longer training period is required.

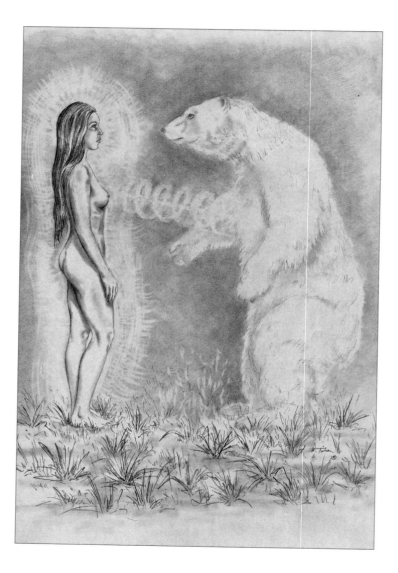

*Working with a power animal helps a person in healing and self-realization*

## Exercise 5: Expanding the Work Together: Dance with a Power Animal

This exercise is only suitable for the Second Degree.

Be sure that you have peace and quiet for the time of the exercise. A room in which you can freely move without bumping into anything or knocking over anything is also necessary. Establish contact with your Inner Child, your Higher Self, and a power animal. Intensify the flow of Reiki energy in every connection. Ask your power animal to come closer to you and show you a dance that is good for you. Then let "it" dance through you. Perceive your body's motions and let yourself go. Nothing bad will happen. The channeled dance will relax your body and possibly permit congested feelings to flow. When the dance has ended or you have had enough, permit yourself at least a 20-minute nap in order to receive the healing effect as completely as possible. Remember to give thanks and carefully end every contact that you have established for this exercise.

## Exercise 6: Channeling a Power Animal

This exercise is only suitable for the Second Degree.

Prepare a microphone and cassette recorder with an empty cassette. Think of a question on a topic that personally effects you and formulate it in writing. It shouldn't be a question that can be answered just with "yes" or "no" or has more than one meaning, such as: "What would happen if I took a vacation in America, France, or Hong Kong in January, March, or August?" An example of an appropriate question would be: "What can I do in order to live the relationship to my partner in the sense of the cosmic order?" or "How should I behave in my profession in relation to the problem (add description of problem) in order to contribute to the benefit of all participants?" Be sure you have peace and quiet during the time of the exercise. As described above, make the Reiki distance contact with your Inner Child, your Higher Self, and a power animal. Intensify the flow of the Reiki energy in all the connections several times. Ask the power animal to answer your question and ask it out loud or in your thoughts exactly like you wrote it down. Now simply speak everything that goes through your mind at the moment onto the tape. Don't censor anything, and don't try to formulate things with a good style. Just say what you perceive. If you wait for something special to happen that you can tell, this exercise won't work! Start talking immediately after you have asked the power animal a question. You'll sense when the answer is complete.

By the way, answers from subtle beings are rarely longwinded. They are used to getting to the point. If you listen to the tape afterwards and think about the information, sort out any possible moral statements, suggestions for improving the world, messages for other people, "do this, don't do that!" instructions, and the like, if there should be any of these. They don't come from a subtle being. They don't make any regulations, are not drearily moralistic, and talk just about you and no one else when you make contact with them, except if someone else has asked you to establish contact for him. It also takes some time for a person to allow himself to become a clear channel for messages from other levels of existence. In my experience, this could happen within three to four days with personal instruction in the scope of a seminar when a person is inexperienced in this field. When learning at home, about three months are realistic, whereby I assume that you will do two or three short exercises a week during this time. If you are strongly involved emotionally with the topic of the question or very interested in the person asking the question and his path in life, experience has shown that it is difficult to channel cleanly. It's better to let a friend who has enough emotional distance work on this topic.

Remember to carefully end every distance contact that you have established for this exercise and to thank each of the exercise partners.

For all the exercises following (and including) Exercise 3a, you can naturally use each method for working with any of the other subtle beings as well. However, based on my experience, I recommend contacts with power animals at the beginning. For the most part, they have been familiar with humans and their character traits for thousands of years. As a result, they are usually patient and don't take things wrong as quickly when they sense that someone simply isn't quite secure enough yet to pay attention to everything but is basically honest, fair, and striving to do everything right. Power animals have many wonderful abilities and carry out many official trips on the Earth as a result of their "jobs." Practically all of them have some humor; however, it can sometimes be quite earthy and eccentric. Some other subtle beings have no understanding of jokes whatsoever. They are nice and want to help, but can't at all understand what it means to play or joke. Later on, you may want to give them some coaching in this direction. If you have the feeling that a subtle partner somehow doesn't know how to go on or is becoming weary, ask whether it would prefer to call another being for this special task, with whom you can work. Remember: none of them can do everything! In addition, systematic, longer work without "breaks for play" can very much irk some power animals. It appears that they aren't made for things like this. Well—who actually is?

# Hidden Knowledge
# in Plants and Minerals

This exercise is only suitable for the Second Degree.

A worthwhile activity is to establish contact with the Higher Self of a type of plant or mineral on a regular basis and let it explain to you what spiritual abilities the representatives of this species possess in relation to healing or personal growth. Always take notes and remember to put your new knowledge to practical use at least once before requesting more information. Otherwise, it's possible that nothing more will come! Shamans and other people who have learned to work with the forces of nature get much for themselves that cannot be found in any book or received from any human teacher. However, never give up your responsibility here either but carefully examine the information that has been channeled to you. This is the spiritual obligation to exercise due care and belongs to the "ABCs" of every light worker of any type.

# Some Examples for Practical Application of Working with Subtle Beings

You can work together with subtle beings in a great variety of ways on even very commonplace problems. Here are some suggestions:

● Make contact with the Higher Self of the house in which you live and give it Reiki on a regular basis. This will considerably increase the quality of life for all the house residents with time and improve the "fate" of the house. Ask the Higher Self if, from its point of view, there is something practical that should be done for the house. You will be astounded by everything that comes out of this. Do your best to translate the suggestions into action. This is also an offering in the sense explained in detail above.

● Make contact with the Higher Selves of mice, rats, flies, ants, or other "pests" if these turn up in your living area on a regular basis. Try to find out why they are there. Sometimes ants come into a house because a natural force that works with them wants to show the inhabitants that there are strong Earth rays there that are good for the ants but very harmful for the people. In such a case, simply setting out ant bait and killing the messengers wouldn't be very meaningful. The existence of "bugs" often shows that the energetic or material structures in an area or building are/have become destructive. Use this as a stimulus for once again creating life-promoting circumstances and you will be acting in the sense of the cosmic laws. The beings that have brought you a message from the spirits will go somewhere else when they are no longer needed at your place—without poison, traps, and swatting.

Sometimes such animals simply need suitable living space for a short time. They are also God's creatures and have their tasks in the world. There is no being with a superfluous existence! Help them in such a case, if you can, and set up a compost pile, a small stack of old wood, or the like in a corner of the garden, for example, or any other suitable place and explain to the Higher Self of this type of animal where there is an appropriate home for its charges. You can also look for somewhere in the neighborhood that would be a good place for these beings to live and where they wouldn't bother anyone, and then tell the corresponding Higher Self where this is. Send it Reiki a number of times so that it can better fulfill its tasks. Remember that strong fear, panic, and stress can extremely disturb the connection to the respective Higher Self and therefore at least prevent it from exerting its influence for a time not only in human beings, but also in animals and plants. If a type of animal crosses your path more frequently for a time, read about the spiritual message of this animal in the corresponding literature. You will often find important messages for yourself in this way. Some shamans also call this a "nature oracle."

⚜ Give the Higher Self of your garden or a forest Reiki on a regular basis and let it advise you in your gardening work. You can also receive information about healing places in nature from it or become informed about certain plants. In time, it can mediate contacts with the devas and elves that work in this piece of nature for you and show you how you can perceive them. Be very careful in how you treat these beings. They are easily frightened and can be injured by vehement imbalanced feelings and insensitive behavior and are therefore frequently afraid of human beings. Is that a surprise for anyone?! Some subtle beings react allergically to iron and steel. In case of doubt, take off everything that is made of these materials before you attempt to make closer contacts with them.

⚜ If you are looking for a new place to live or a new job, in addition to the customary methods of evaluation you can also establish a connection with the respectively responsible Higher Self and let yourself be advised as to whether this place is suitable for you.

⚜ Bring the blessing of the creative power into your property by giving the Higher Self of your car Reiki now and then, for example. In the old days, this was something quite common. The ritualistic christening of ships still reminds us of this and in some areas, a priest is called even today in order to bless tools, residences, animals, and the like. Giving a Higher Self Reiki has the same meaning as this type of blessing.

- Learn something about nature and the laws according to which it functions at the source: the Higher Self of a plant, an animal, or a mineral.
- Establish contact with the Higher Self of the weather in an area where you are at the moment. Send it Reiki and ask it to create a harmonious climate, if this is in the sense of the cosmic order.
- Establish contact with the Higher Self of a stream and feel your way into it, draw a picture of it, or dance with it.

As you will notice, there is a vast quantity of exciting experiments. And this is just the beginning, the basic level of Rainbow Reiki...

# CHAPTER FIVE

# Rainbow Reiki and Energy Work with Power Places

## General Information on Power Places

Every place, every being, and every material object has a field of force that is woven around it from many different energies in a more or less solid structure. Each of these emanation patterns is solid in relation to the essence of its identity, which is what gives a part of the Creation its unique nature. The emanation is changeable because there are formative relationships with other things and beings that develop, shift, or otherwise transform the parts of the field. Patterns from the outside can enter into the field of force, blend into it, and also again leave it in part or completely at a given time. Modifications in the energy field of a place, object, or being[28] can also occur because of fluctuations in the strength of the overall emanation or the emanation of certain areas.

The energetic fields (auras) of places, beings, or objects basically enter into a relationship with each other on the various qualitative levels when:

a. strong emotions or other energetic interactions of a qualitative or quantitative sort currently exist in relation to the others

b. a basis of communication adequately accessible to both for a conscious and differentiated, as well as unconscious, exchange is found.

How strong the contact and the exchange associated with it is depends on the receptivity of the partner in the relationship and the strength of the emanation of their energy fields.

If I relate these statements to dealing with power places, this means that every place is basically a power place in the larger sense of the word. However, this doesn't apply to every person at any given time and in any way, varying greatly in intensity and quality. In other words, if you feel particularly well in the proximity of a

---

[28] From the spiritual perspective, these three manifestation forms of the divine Creation cannot necessarily be distinctly separated from each other.

large, old tree or a pilgrimage site, this doesn't mean that every other person will have the same experiences at these places. Often the special power of a place can only be experienced when the receptivity for subtle impressions is significantly increased through a learning process, meaning that the basis for communication with other parts of the world is expanded. In the narrower sense, power places are something that gives *you* power, convey important knowledge, or influence you in a way that is positive in the overall sense. Some places will only be important for you at certain times or even just once in your life. Others can accompany you for a long time, perhaps as long as you are on this plane. Such power places can also give you support in difficult times and teach you to successfully get through the valleys in life and properly enjoy the mountain tops. These great teachers have frequently helped many people and, in a certain respect, they are also there for this purpose. On the other hand, you can also give them important help in exchange by offering them Reiki, staying in contact with them on a regular basis, and doing other important things for them that are enjoyable for you. When you work with it in such a way, a place of power can continue to grow and receive more possibilities of helping and healing.

If you increasingly develop the ability within you to listen, look, and deeply open yourself for what surrounds you, you will soon notice that there are many power places for you in your immediate environment and that they possess varying attributes. With time you will better perceive their individuality and learn to sense their consciousness and messages. Their needs and talents will be increasingly revealed to you. This will cause profound possibilities of being and working together to open up for you. This chapter should help you to expand these special abilities and put them to good use. Reiki will pave the way for you and create the possibilities of contact with power places, their Higher Selves, and the subtle beings connected with these places, the development of which requires years of intensive training to accomplish in another manner for most people.

There is much to discover and learn. The best place to have the first experiences with power places is in God's open countryside.

# The Differing Qualities of Power Places

When you walk through the landscape, time and again you will come across places that direct attention to themselves and have something "special" about them. If you stop at such a place for some time, it can easily happen that you get into a peculiar, enraptured mood. Some people have discovered such a lovely spot of earth at some point and then visit it time and again in order to tank energy, clear their minds, or get relief for emotional or physical complaints. As an example, a Reiki friend told me that he goes back to a certain tree over and over again in order to soothe his heart complaints. The healing influence of the tree on him was so intensive that it could even be clearly proved in a long-term ECG[29].

If a certain place has a harmonizing, animating, or even consciousness-expanding effect on people, it is called a *positive power place*. There are also power places with an emanation or characteristic that burdens human beings. Here accidents, diseases, imbalanced emotional states, or crimes occur more frequently than in other places. These are *negative power places*. It is not always possible to clearly classify a place in a specific category, negative or positive. Frequently, just certain people are influenced by one type of effect. In the same respect, not everyone necessarily reacts at all to the emanation of a certain power place.

Many power places of both types are generally known. However, the majority of power places tend to lead a secluded existence. This is not necessarily because they are less capable of being effective, but because they are not perceived by human beings or even because they are not considered to be so important. So they more or less slumber and lie dormant, waiting for someone to come who is willing to work with them, for a person to come to them who has learned to listen to their fine voices and take their messages seriously.

When you have carefully worked through this chapter, you will be able to recognize power places, understand their different abilities, and communicate with them. It will also be possible for you, as it was for the people of ancient times who were close to nature, to create new power places under certain preconditions, awaken those that are asleep, activate their fallow abilities, and meaningfully deal with them in a variety of ways.

You can successfully use a series of the methods presented in this chapter with the First Reiki Degree. However, for others you will definitely need the Second Degree. A further prerequisite is that you have read through the previous chapter about approaching subtle beings, tried out the introductory exercises, and have understood the basics for working with subtle beings before you start the practical work with power places described here.

---

[29] This is a procedure in which a small electronic measuring instrument is worn by a heart patient for a longer period of time so that more values are available for medical evaluation of the heart's condition.

# Various Categories of Power Places

There are many different types of power places with a strong emanation and particularly prominent possibilities of effectiveness. I have listed them for you in this section and described their special qualities in detail. Take a good look at all of this and then find examples from your own experience for each category so that you have "partners" for the exercises explained below.

## I. Power places created by human beings

All places that have been consciously or unconsciously accentuated in the significance of their emanation and/or possibilities of effectiveness fall into this category.

### a. Power places in which like-minded people frequently have come together

If, for example, people come together in a hall time and again in order to celebrate, in time the room will be so "drenched" in vibrations of the same type that it begins to reflect these energetic impressions on various levels after having achieved a certain degree of charging. This is practical when people come together there whose plans are supported by the emanation. In *dojos*, the traditional Japanese exercise rooms for fighting arts, meditation, or other consciousness-expanding activities, it is very important that a certain mental attitude is cultivated. In time, every person who enters the room will receive help in his work and the development of his personality that should not be underestimated through the reflection of the place.

### b. Power places in which strong emotions have often been released

One negative example is the atmosphere of medieval torture chambers, which still send a very unpleasant shudder down most visitors' backs. In the positive sense, you can perceive an emanation in a playroom that happy children have used for years, which can even prompt some adults to romp around and play there.

### c. Power places in which energy work has been done on a regular basis

Old altars, the lodge houses of the Freemasons or other societies in which energy work has been performed for a long time, as well as temples, holy groves, and churches receive a typical emanation clearly differentiating them from other places not only in intensity but also type through magical, shamanistic, or mystic practices during the course of the years.

### d. Power places that are characterized by special architectural, geometric, or material features

Some buildings have been consciously or unconsciously designed and built from materials that have the effect of a type of convex lens for subtle vibrations of a certain sort. The *orgon accumulators* invented by *Wilhelm Reich*, the Austrian psychiatrist and natural scientist, are an example of this. As a result of the alternating ordering of organic and inorganic materials, they collect certain subtle energies through the one side and emit them in a bundled manner on the other side.

### e. Power places that have received their special emanation through nuclear, electromagnetic, or electrical facilities

Every nuclear reactor, every electrical transformer facility, and every television tower represents a power place. Through the strong electrical, electromagnetic, and/or nuclear energies that collect and move here, there is an extensive interaction with subtle vibrations. The principle of reciprocal influence of subtle and conventional-physical energies behind this is applied, for example, by Kirlian photography in which the characteristic interactions of an electrical high-voltage field with the aura of a living being can be photographed.

The reciprocal influence and the powers behind it are not basically negative. They can also be used for healing purposes if the necessary knowledge exists. However, there are practically always negative effects on the body and mind when the energies are too strong and/or appear in a form that is too chaotic. Since subtle conditions and their effects on living beings are not yet taken into consideration in the construction methods for large-scale electrical, electromagnetic, or nuclear facilities, the power places mentioned under this point are not places with which you should necessarily establish physical or subtle contact. It's not much fun, although it will not directly cause harm if you adhere to the Reiki methods. Nevertheless, the connection can cause a *great deal* of emotional confusion for you.

## II. Power places created by subtle beings

This category of power places also has an "artificial" origin. Subtle beings of all types build energetic structures on their home plane of existence and sometimes also on our own for a great variety of purposes and anchor them on places that appear suitable to them because of their natural state. Strongly charged, differentiated subtle-energetic structures always emanate into other levels of existence and may possibly trigger reactions in a variety of other ways on the plane where the basic structure exists. Rituals, amulets, and other material power objects, for example, function according to this principle.

### a. Contact places

There is a type of bridge from one plane of existence to another or others. Very few of them permit a complete material crossing into another dimension under certain conditions, such as specific areas in the Bermuda Triangle, for example. For the most part, they tend to create a communicative connection. They strengthen the abilities of beings to perceive other levels of the Creation with their senses, receive messages from them, and send messages there themselves. Many stone circles, temples, and grave mounds have been built on such places. I have listed this type of power place under the category "created by subtle beings" because these have been the builders in most cases. However, human beings are basically capable of manifesting such an energy structure, even if some training and experience, as well as patience and good connections to the spirits, are required for this purpose.

### b. Refuges

When subtle beings like angels or spiritual teachers are active on our plane, without incarnating in the material sense, they need a type of foothold that makes it possible for them to stay and have an effect here without greater efforts on their part. These great helpers are usually not constantly bound to one place, yet it represents an important source of strength for them and their possibilities of effectiveness are often most comprehensive there. In earlier times, people frequently built temples or altars at these sites and visited them when they needed extensive spiritual support. The refuges are well-suited for people to take a rest at the major crossroads of their path in life, find advice and understanding, and become clearer about the meaning and purpose of their existence.

### c. Subtle energy machines

There is an entire series of possibilities for collecting subtle energies, meaningfully structuring and lastingly stabilizing them, and permitting them to be effective for certain tasks. Beings of the subtle dimension, as well as individual human beings, master the art of building and using such facilities. In ancient times, these machines were used to heal and influence the climate, as well as help animals, plants, people, and subtle beings live in harmony with each other even in difficult situations or be able to communicate with each other over great distances. The possibilities for using such facilities are enormously versatile. In our times, most of these are "sleeping" and waiting in the "stand-by" mode to once again be awakened and put to use.

### d. Power places with special tasks

Even today, native peoples are familiar with places that are sought out for specific purposes such as harvest festivals, blessing of the kill, initiation of healers or social leaders, or preparation of adolescents for introduction into the world of adults. At these places there are often possibilities for contacting subtle teacher beings, who consider their tasks to be working together with human beings in a certain area. Places that are used to this effect can also belong to other categories.

## III. Natural power places

Among these are all places that represent special concentration points of the subtle flow of energy on the Earth. Just like human beings, the Earth also has nerve paths, meridians (as they are described in traditional Chinese medicine), chakras, and acupuncture points. She has sensory organs, such as the trees that grow on her body, and a consciousness, which does differ greatly from its human counterpart. However, since the Earth is a being of this plane of existence representing the life basis for all other creatures on this planet, she is strongly connected with her "children" in a certain way. In the shamanistic sweat-lodge rituals or other healing applications of the Earth energy, the connection of a human being to the Great Mother, as the Earth is also called by native peoples and traditional healers, is used for strengthening purposes and the harmonization of deep fears, psychosomatic afflictions, and life crises of all types. The power of the Earth is enormous. If, perhaps one day, our society once again recollects that we human beings are her children and she is not our slave, we will have a good chance of healing the environmental damages of the past few decades.

### a. Cliffs

Cliffs are the bones of the Earth. A cliff is a good place to let inner stability grow. Here you can learn how you can become strong enough, give your life meaning and happiness, master difficult, strenuous situations, and come to rest within yourself. Cliffs have differing powers, according to where they are located, what type of rock they are composed of, and possibly who works with them from the subtle planes.

### b. Caves

Among other things, you can find protection, basic trust, and a feeling of security in a cave. This is the Great Mother's womb. Connected with certain rituals that awaken the healing power of the Earth, the visit to a cave can free you from blocks that can hardly be dissolved in any other way. Sometimes this is like a snake shedding its skin, a person goes bent by worry into a cave and after the ritual is over, appears radiant, liberated, and as if he were reborn from the body of the Great Mother. Some native peoples also use cave rituals to prepare themselves for the transition into a new phase of life. Caves are particularly well-suited (as are the corresponding sweat lodges) to developing and strengthening the loving, harmonious spirit of community. Whether good relationships between people alone or between them and their environment are concerned, a cave can bring unity into the diversity and free from separation. This is how the strong healing effect of cave rituals on physical or emotional imbalances based on suppression or the separation of certain parts of a human being's personality can be explained.

### c. Trees and holy groves

Trees are important parts of the sensory organs, the memory, and the detoxification organs of the Earth. Old trees have special abilities. Their wisdom, which has grown through many decades, and their experience can give us human beings special knowledge to put us in the position of once again bringing our life into harmony with nature. Like gigantic antennas, their mighty crowns (still) reach up to the heavens, from which they receive many types of energies. Their leaves are like highly sensitive antennas, suited for responding to almost any kind of vibrations. Large trees have become increasingly few in number, the rain forests are systematically or even just thoughtlessly cut down, many wonderful forms of life—plants and animals—are disappearing with them. I don't know if we human beings can comprehend on time what we are doing to ourselves and our environment with this "clear-cutting" throughout the world. But I hope we will. In addition to political commitment, a change in personal behavior, and enlightenment work such as the Rainbow Reiki energy work can provide an important contribution to maintaining our mutual basis for life. After you have visited a tree on the subtle level, spoken with it, and experienced its friendliness and wisdom, you will treat plant life in a different way. We can make Reiki available to the forests so that they can better survive the high degree of strain in our age, and we can support the subtle beings responsible for the plants, the devas and elves in the mastering of their tasks with our possibilities.

## d. Clearings
If clearings are formed naturally, the reason may be a strongly imbalanced Earth emanation, which is basically nothing "evil" but a type of detoxification place or even an energy-reception point of high capacity. Places of this type are not suited for people to stay at for a longer period of time. But they can also represent one of the many Earth chakras. In this case, the clearing will be full of life and practically invite you to stay there. Several hours of dreaming to yourself there can bring your body, mind, and soul back into harmony and help reinstate the proper, healthy relationship between relaxation and performance in life. Please note: the Earth's chakras can also be found in places other than natural clearings (see below under g.). Subtle beings like to meet in clearings at certain times.

## e. Bodies of water
Medicinal springs still play a great role in our times. Many baths and spa facilities are grouped around springs whose healing power has sometimes been known and valued for centuries. However, modern spa doctors are more concerned about certain contents and their effects on the metabolism in the biological-chemical sense. Yet, the water of some wells has much more to offer. It's no coincidence that sagas, fairy-tales, and legends are centered on bodies of water in general and springs in particular. For the Earth, water is a means of solution and transportation that receives all types of energies and substances in endless natural rhythms when they have become *superfluous* in one place and takes them to places where there is still an unfulfilled need for them. Some subtle beings like to establish their refuges at springs, ponds, or watercourses. Water generally promotes communication. (Think of drinks at celebrations and parties.) In society, as well as in the body of the individual, it permits information to flow more easily. The flow of emotions also has a strong affinity to water. In traditional Chinese medicine, a correlation between the two was already established centuries ago. Perhaps this is why vacation spots "on the water" are so popular because it's easier here to get the vital forces constricted by everyday life flowing again.

## f. Mountains
The Earth, the Great Mother, establishes connect with the sky, the Great Father, through the mountains. This is why mountain tops are particularly suited for achieving clarity, for inspiration and the pro-

motion of creative power, as well as strengthening individuality, self-confidence, and self-respect. For some Indian tribes it is still common today to request the personal vision, an ideal for the meaning and goal of one's own path in life, within the scope of a special ritual called *vision quest* from the powers of the heavens on the top of a mountain or a plateau. If you become lost in the jungle of your everyday life, you can help yourself by going to the mountains and coming closer to their power on long walks there. With their help, you can once again attain a better perspective. Difficulties are again put into the proper proportions in comparison to pleasant experiences, and some whales turn into guppies.

Since earliest times, certain mountains have been considered holy. Whoever has made the effort of hiking through the mountain world of the Alps, for example, and felt their powerful emanation, will be able to confirm this from his own experience. In Europe, particularly the Celts often maintained altars, temples, and spiritual centers on mountains, hills, and cliffs in order to come closer to their gods. The ancient Greeks were convinced that Olympus—a high mountain located in Greece—was the home of their gods. Even today, the names of many rises in the countryside give evidence of their earlier spiritual tasks.

### g. Earth chakras and Earth acupuncture points
Just like human beings, animals, and plants, the Earth also has a subtle energy system. As a result, there are Earth chakras that organize and represent the life functions of our planet on the energetic level; there are communication channels (meridians) that connect these energy centers with each other and naturally also points on these conductive paths that have a function for the Earth similar to that of acupuncture points for the human body. The entire body of the Earth is crossed by these energy networks and intersecting points. When subtle vibrations concentrated in one place are sucked into the Earth, this is called a negative Earth-emanation zone. The pendulum usually shows a counterclockwise direction here. Human beings and many animals experience health disorders more quickly than in other places. Chronic and degenerative imbalances are promoted here in particular. Constant tiredness, fatigue, and a weakening of the immune system can be the consequences. If energy is transported out of the Earth to a more extensive degree, it is usually a so-called positive Earth-emanation zone. A pendulum will normally swing clockwise. It is not easy to sleep or generally achieve a state of rest here. Nervousness, irritability, and restlessness will occur after some time.

92

# How You Can Meaningfully Work with Power Places

When working with power places it is important to approach them in a way that permits you to feel their individuality and always adequate time for you to become accustomed to their emanation, always offering a different way of establishing contact. Practically every power place likes to work with human beings if they don't trample on it in a disrespectful, egoistic, and insensitive manner. There is a big difference between whether you just want to go for a walk in lovely surroundings or if you approach a power place with the intention of any type of energetic work. When you go for a walk, you only have to be concerned with the matters of environmental protection that are quite obvious in our times such as: not making a lot of noise and startling the animals, not pulling plants out of the ground, and not leaving any garbage in the middle of nature. There is no power place and no subtle being that will be angry with you if you simply want to enjoy the natural environment. But if you want healing, knowledge, help in solving problems or developing your personality, and the like, you should stick to the rules for establishing contact. You will learn how to approach a power place in a competent way in the next section. Read through it carefully and follow these rules, which have been valid and functioning for millennia. Then you will achieve the best results in your work with power places. It is thoroughly possible to even establish contact with power places and maintain a relationship satisfactory to both sides using the First Degree. I have described the methods necessary for this purpose under the heading "If you have been initiated into the First Degree." The higher level of work with power places will open up for you on the Reiki path through the Second Degree. You will find the details on this under the heading "If you have been initiated into the Second Degree."

# Basic Exercises for Power-Place Work

With some simple exercises, you can develop your abilities of perceiving power places and communicating with them.

### Exercise 1: Finding positive and negative Earth-emanation zones in your living space

For this exercise, you need about a half hour. Be sure you have peace and quiet so that you can open up to this new type of perception without being disturbed. If you have been initiated into the First Degree, give yourself about 10 minutes of Reiki on the first and second major chakras.[30] These two energy center are not the Inner Child, but it can be indirectly strengthened through them. This is how you can show that you want to have contact with it and are there for it.

If you have been initiated into the Second Degree, establish contact with your Inner Child through distance Reiki. For this purpose, use the distance-treatment signs and the energy-intensification signs, as well as the corresponding mantras you have learned, and clearly direct the Reiki by calling the "Inner Child of (your first and last name)." Turn your hands away from your body and don't try to visualize your Inner Child. Intensify the flow of Reiki a number of times and wait to see what happens. After several minutes, request your Inner Child to assist you in your following plans, even if it hasn't made itself noticeable in a spectacular way. If you correctly establish contact as described here, it will receive your request.

The Inner Child is the part of you that controls the subtle senses and possibilities of action. If you strengthen it through indirect offerings of Reiki (First Degree) or through a direct Reiki treatment (distance contact), it can more effectively apply its abilities and better communicate with you. Don't expect your Inner Child to speak to you in words. Its way of communicating is through images, physical sensations, and other sensory perceptions. It doesn't think in a logical-rational manner, but in patterns, symbols, and comprehensive correlations. It doesn't master its tasks through work, but by playing creatively.

Now close your eyes and request that you can feel a place that is good for you in the room where you are. Without giving it much thought, go to this place. Stay there for about 10 minutes. Perceive the changes that happen in your physical sensations, your emotions, and your mind when you are there. Don't expect anything in particular so you won't have a filter in front of your senses. Also take perceptions seriously that are less than spectacular. Don't try to interpret them, just experience them.

Next, ask your Inner Child to show you another place in the room that's not good for you. Go to this spot, but only stay as long as you need to in order to perceive the difference to your "little power place" where you previously were. Then go back to the place where you felt good for a while in order to once again become harmonized. Don't forget to take leave of the contact if you have used a Second Degree connection.

---

[30]See the Appendix "A Brief Explanation of the Chakras" for the position of the major chakras.

You can integrate this little exercise into your everyday life with great benefit to yourself. Look for places to work and rest that support you and avoid places that weaken your strength as much as possible. The more you do this, the easier it will be for you. With time, your perception will become refined and you will increasingly have the ability to differentiate between the various emanations of the Earth and their greater and lesser intensity. If the subtle impressions should become too much for you at some point, then breath calmly and deeply into your lower belly, just below your navel, for about 15 minutes or longer. This is where your hara, a type of collecting place for energies, is located. If you focus your attention on this spot (the exact location of which you don't need to know down to the millimeter in order to work with it effectively) for a longer period of time, you will quickly be with yourself. You will then find inner peace and be able to collect yourself. Resting within oneself by shifting the attention to the hara is an important technique for dealing with subtle energy work with a balanced approach in the long run. Observe animals and their favorite spots with this new type of perception. Some animals like emanation qualities that are similar to those you prefer, and others practically look for negative vibrations. Ants, for example, like to build their nests in places with Earth radiation harmful to human beings. Cats also often lie on zones that have a negative effect on people and most other mammals. However, in contrast to ants and many other insects, they are not at home there in the direct sense because they need these vibrations. Their coat just insulates them against the energy flow there, and when they want to be alone, they make use of this ability. Then most other animals won't disturb them when they rest on such a spot.

## Exercise 2: Drawing a power place

Take some colored pencils and a drawing block. Look for an old tree or some other power place. Feel your way into its emanation with the senses trained by the first exercise.

If you have the First Degree, give yourself about 15 minutes of Reiki on your first and second major chakras while doing this.

If you have the Second Degree, establish contact, as described in the first exercise—with your Inner Child. Then make distance contact with the Higher Self of this place by using the distance-contact symbol, the energy-intensification symbol, and the corresponding mantras, as you learned to do in your Second-Degree training. Then direct the flow of Reiki energy by clearly calling the "Higher Self of this power place (add the name of the place, if possible)" three times. Intensify the flow of Reiki a number of times.

For both degrees: feel your way into what is happening for a while. Then, without giving it any thought, take one of the pencils and start to draw a picture. Let it happen. You will feel when it is done. Then give thanks and end the contact with the Second Degree or first put your hands on your heart for a moment and then on the Earth close to the power place, giving thanks, if you have been initiated into the First Degree.

The exercise "drawing power-place pictures" will develop your senses and your intuitive understanding of subtle messages even further than you have already experienced in the previous chapter with a similar exercise. Do this on a regular basis, at least once or twice a week for a longer period of time. It is very important that you don't think about what you want to draw and don't try to control the process that creates the picture with your will. Only when the rational mind withdraws can your subtle perceptions be correctly translated through your Inner Child, which controls your body. A meditative calmness and an opening of the self is what occurs in the process. Let it happen—resonate with it without doing anything or having to control anything.

Meditate on your work of art that has been created in this way every day for several minutes by looking at one of the pictures and simply letting your thoughts flow freely. If you notice that you are thinking about something completely different, look at the picture again and wait to see what associations arise. This is particularly intense before you go to sleep. Pay attention to your dreams!

When you have carried out both of these exercises a number of times, you should be well-prepared to open up more to power places and their emanations, messages, and special abilities. Unfortunately, I can't tell you exactly how long you will need for this within the scope of a book. You may need a few weeks or possible even a few months in order to expand your subtle perception. You will sense whether or not you are ready. Haste and impatience only cause harm. Take your time. The path is important.

## Exercise 3: Selecting and approaching a power place

For the further exercises, you will need a power place with a greater capacity such as a large, old tree, a stone circle from the megalith culture, a holy mountain, or some other cult site. Before you get closer to this place:

—If you have been initiated into the First Degree, give yourself about 15 minutes of Reiki on the 1st and 2nd major chakra and then about 5 minutes of Reiki on the 6th chakra (third eye) and the 4th chakra (heart center).

—If you have been initiated into the Second Degree, give your Inner Child Reiki through the distance contact, as described in Exercise 1. Now additionally establish a Reiki contact to your Higher Self through distance contact by using the distance-treatment symbol and the energy-intensification symbol, as well as the corresponding mantras, as you have learned to do. Clearly direct the flow of the Reiki energy by using calling the "Higher Self of (add your first and last name)". Turn the palms of your hands away from your body and don't expect anything in particular. Above all, don't try to imagine a picture of your Higher Self. If you do so, it will limit its possibilities of communicating with you or helping you in some other way. Let things happen as they want to happen.

For both degrees: Ask your Higher Self and your Inner Child in your thoughts or out loud for their support and their protection in your plan of establishing contact with the chosen power place. Only take leave of this Second-Degree distance contact when you have again left the power place at the end of your work and are out of its area of emanation area. If you have been initiated into the First Degree, take leave at the end of the power-place work and give thanks. Now feel your way into what has changed for a moment. Don't expect anything spectacular. Practical energy work isn't necessarily like what you have seen in fantasy films at first... Now approach the center of the power place.

# Recognizing and Learning to Use the Various Working Areas of a Power Place

Every larger place of power has various zones, which respectively perceive certain functions in the contact with the others. Within this, I differentiate between the following:

### The emanation boundary

Here is the outer boundary of the effective area of a power place. There are frequently watercourses, trenches, field borders, paths, or a different type of vegetation there where the invisible boundary of the immediate emanation of a power place runs. When you have crossed these lines and adjusted yourself to the subtle perceptions, you will suddenly notice a distinctly stronger intensity in the emanation of the power place. Go back and forth a few times in order to become more certain in the perception of the emanation boundary. The distance of this boundary from the center of the power place will vary. For an old tree, it could possibly be about 100 meters or less. When I visited the ashram[31] of Sathya Sai Baba[32] in the vicinity of the Indian city of Bangladore, I felt the emanation boundary in a clear increase of a strong, light vibration already at a distance of more than 20 kilometers. In some cases, the emanation boundary of a power place is flexible. It can shift in connection with the moon cycles or seasons, for example.

If you have reached the emanation boundary, make contact with the Higher Self of this place as in Exercise 2, if you have been initiated into the Second Degree. If you have been initiated into the First Degree, simply feel your way into your surroundings for a moment and put your hands on the area of your heart.

For both degrees, say the following in your thoughts or out loud:

*I come to you as an unhealthy person and request healing. I come to you as an ignorant person and ask for teaching. I come to you as a helpless person and ask for support and protection. I come to you as a powerless person and ask for power in order to better serve. In return for your help, I offer you Reiki.*

Be clear about the meaning of this way of addressing the place and think about it time and again before you make deeper contact with a place of power. Then use the energy-intensification of the Second Degree in distance contact with the Higher Self of the place or place your hands on the Earth for several minutes if you have the First Degree.

Now it's time to move closer to the center of the power place.

### The inner area

When you have gone a bit further, you will again feel a distinct increase in the emanation of the place. Try to perceive the boundary as precisely as you can, take some steps back and forth and pay attention to the change that results. Then finally go into the inner area and use some further intensification signs in order to let even more Reiki flow to the Higher Self of the place or, if you have been initiated into the First Degree, again place your hands on the Earth for several minutes so that Reiki can flow to the power place. Open yourself for what is happening. It could be that the guardian of the place is now

---

[31] An ashram is a place of spiritual work, maintained by a spiritual teacher.
[32] Sathya Sai Baba is a saint born in India and spiritual teacher active throughout the world.

already willing to start working with you, even if you haven't expressed a concrete wish yet. You can perhaps notice this in a flowing and streaming, a feeling of warmth or coldness. Blocked feelings can rise within you quite unexpectedly and want to express themselves in physical terms. Let this happen. This is among the gifts from a power place that it frees you from blocks in order to create space for a new liveliness within you.

### The path of opening up/letting go

The more you now approach the center of the emanation, the most important it becomes for the success of the power-place work that you open up. Observe the plants, listen to the rushing of the wind and the voices of the animals. Surrender yourself to the mood of this special area and believe in your feelings. It's completely normal for you to feel insecurity or fear or for your rational mind to constantly rebel and try to make it clear to you that what you are doing is nonsense. Be inside your own feelings and be critical, and let new experiences happen. Then you have the best precondition for close work with a power place on the basis of equality.

Later, when you have finished the work, if possible, return on the same path that you came on and use it to achieve an inner distance from the power place and once again become more conscious of the everyday human world. Direct your attention to areas and events outside of the emanation area. Give thanks in your mind or out loud for what you have received and request that you will once again be accepted there when it is time for you to return. The path of opening up/letting go is responsible for the cleansing of your energy field. When you come, you will be freed of many vibrations that could have hindered you from opening up to the power place. When you go, the power place helps you once again structure your aura in the way required for the everyday world of human beings.

But first go back into the vibration of the place once again.

### The place of greeting

Let yourself be led by the guardian of the place, who now has become more familiar with you, to a suitable place of greeting for you. Request guidance in your mind or quietly out loud and then walk around, without thinking much about it, until you have the feeling you should stop. Stop at this spot. You can sit down, lie down, or even remain standing. It isn't important for what now will happen. If you have been initiated into the Second Degree, intensify the flow of the Reiki energy in the distance contact a number of times. In the First Degree, place one hand on your heart and the other on the Earth. Now request acceptance. It will take some minutes, sometimes perhaps even more than a half hour, before the guardian of the power place has increased and modified your vibration to the point that it has largely been adapted to its own. This process is necessary to improve the communication between the two of you and open up more possibilities for the power place to help you. It may be necessary to visit the same place a number of times until your vibration can be intensified and structured in the manner required for a more complex working relationship without doing any harm to you. Be patient if this is the case. Alone through this increasing adaptation, completely new areas will open up to you. Your mind will become clearer, your senses will become sharper, and, if you permit it, rising feelings will be physically expressed and many blocks that hinder the flow of your vital energies will be dissolved. Many people have reported that after this attunement—please don't confuse this with an initiation—they were able to perceive colors, sounds, smells, and physical sensations in a new, often previously unknown intensity and clarity. It is possible that you will get a bit of a queasy feeling in your stomach or become slightly dizzy during an attunement procedure. Perhaps you will also begin to laugh or suddenly feel like you are safe and sound in God's trouser pocket. If you are well-attuned to a power place, you might possibly see dancing elves, hear the song of the flowers and trees, and be able to observe dwarfs. Be respectful and don't impose yourself. Wait until a subtle being approaches you and establishes contact with you on its own.[33]

If you should now want to shut this book because you possibly believe there is something missing in terms of my mental health, please wait just one more moment and give me and you a chance. Don't believe anything I say. Carefully try out what I have explained here and you will probably soon tell your best friends, when you are alone together, something about the wonderful, strange, and yet somehow so deeply familiar experiences that you have had.

It is once again time for human beings and the beings of the subtle world, of nature, and the elements to come together in peace. The Age of Aquarius is beginning, and many things will be different—it will be a bit like earlier days in ancient times, of which the fairytales tell so much. We usually no longer believe in this as adults. Yet, you can now experience it yourself and help others have similar experiences. Take the first step. Have faith in yourself. The powers of light and love will help you because they have a great interest in this world once again becoming more intact.

---

[33] Remember to carefully remove everything made of iron or steel before you enter into closer contact with one of these beings.

## Places with special functions within
### the working area of the power place

When the attunement has ended, request out loud or in your thoughts that the power place help you in solving one of your important personal problems or, if you currently have nothing urgent on your mind, simply request its support in developing your own ability to be happy. Then ask to be shown a spot suitable for your plan. Walk on, without thinking much about it, until you have the feeling that you should stop. Now let the power place work with you. Nothing bad will happen to you in the objective sense, yet it is possible that you will feel emotional or physical pain for a short time. This indicates that blocks are being dissolved and firmly-held energies are starting to flow. The more you open up for this, the more honest you are, the deeper the help of the power place can work within you. If it becomes too much for you, tell this out loud or mentally to the guardian of the place. It will respect your decision. Remember that Rome wasn't built in one day either. Extensive changes need time. Often you will only be deeply relaxed, perhaps even fall asleep and wake up refreshed and somehow more clear and alive as a result of its intervention. You will only later discover some results in your everyday life.

It can be very interesting if you examine the power place with a pendulum and determine which of its areas have a special effect on your chakras or meridians. But don't get hung up on such research results. In their many different qualities, the subtle energies are far from being researched extensively enough by human beings in order for us to truly be able to understand everything that happens at a power place. We can hardly approach this with our rational minds. But this is also great fun and very exciting, and it will expand your world view.

If you would like to have a present for a friend blessed by a power place, want to have a couple relationship confirmed in a spiritual manner, or would like to celebrate the party of the century, request the guardian of the place to give you information on the spot most suitable for the respective purpose, for its help and hospitality. The parties created in this manner will be an unforgettable experience for you and possible others who participate.

### The place to take leave

If you have the feeling that the guardian of the place would like to end the work with you or if you yourself would like to stop, give thanks for what you have received. Then request a place in which you can complete your attunement to the "normal" vibrational level. Look for it intuitively, as you now are perhaps used to doing, without giving it much thought. If you have been initiated into the Second Degree, intensify the flow of the Reiki energy in the distance contact a number of times. In the First Degree, place one hand on your heart and the other on the Earth. Now request that you once again be attuned to your everyday vibration. Wait a bit until you have the feeling that you are again "more in reality" or that the process has been completed. Then go slowly and consciously the "path of opening up/letting go" and gradually detach your attention from the emanation of the power place. When you are on the boundary of the inner area, take leave from the Higher Self of the power place, as you have learned to do if you have been initiated into the First Degree. Give thanks for its attention and ask to be permitted to come to it again. If you have been initiated into the First Degree, place one hand on your heart and the other on the Earth, give thanks, and also ask to be accepted again for following visits. Take leave from your Inner Child and your own Higher Self, if you have been in contact with them through the Second Degree, only when you are on the emanation boundary. In the First Degree, put your hands together in front of your heart, simply give thanks, bow, and feel within yourself for a moment.

After you have read this section, you are now familiar with a complete and diverse basic program of power-place work with Rainbow Reiki. There are naturally many, many other things you could do in connection with power places, but you should first, in as far as this is possible for you, do practical work with the exercises described here and gather experiences. Much will be taught to you by the power places themselves. For other things you may need human teachers. You will find them when the time is really right and you are willing to learn.

# Gifts You Can Receive
# from a Power Place

You can receive a series of energetic or even material types of gifts from power places. They can be deep mystical experiences, sudden insights, healings, knowledge, as well as leaves, stones, sand, branches, and similar tangible things. Sometimes the powers of a place ask you to bring drawing materials with you on your next visit because they would like to put a picture on paper through you. Perhaps you will have the desire to sing or dance while at a power place. Go ahead and do it, even if you have a strange feeling about it at first. Many people have had wonderful, healing experiences in this manner. When I need a power song, a mantra, a dance or drum ritual for my work or for myself privately, I frequently visit power places that I have been familiar with for a long time, attune myself to them, explain my plans to them, and request that they help me. As a result, I have learned much that has given joy to myself and others, as well as being very useful.

Be very careful about *never* cutting or tearing anything from living trees or other plants. Don't pick any flowers and don't pull out any plants. Only take a pebble or any other stone with you if it has literally been placed before your feet, and still ask in addition if it is for you and to be taken with you. In no case should you knock material out of a cliff or cave. You can take anything that has fallen off, but don't forget to give thanks for it and, in First Degree give Reiki to the Earth of the power place or have an extra portion of universal life energy sent to the Higher Self of the place with the Second Degree distance contact through the intensification technique as an exchange.

Treat the natural powers and subtle beings in general and places of power in particular with respect, attention, thankfulness, and modesty. Then you will have wonderful experiences with them and receive fantastic presents.

# Cross-Linking Power Places
# with Each Other

When you have done power-place work for a longer period of time, it can happen that one of these places requests you to help it repair the Earth's communication lines that have been torn apart. Then you should, for example, take a stone, the water from a spring, plant

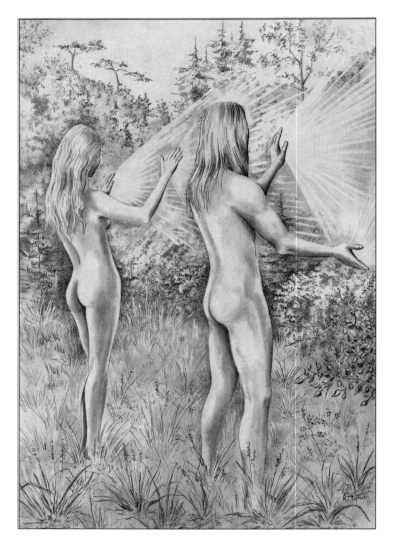

*Holistic environmental protection also includes energy work*

seeds like acorns or chestnuts, or something else from one place and bring it to another power place. These things are needed to set up new transmission and reception stations for the transference of subtle information and power. With this, you can provide a very great service for the beings responsible for reestablishing harmony in our world. The more and the better the energy networks between the subtle centers of Mother Earth are connected, the more effectively the diverse types of environmental damage in our time can be headed off and perhaps even repaired at some point. Power places of all types function better when they are connected with others and in loving company. Just like human beings.

## How You Can Set Up a Power Place

At the conclusion of this chapter, there is still one special bonus for you. However, you can only carry it out if you have been initiated into the Second Reiki Degree. Now you can learn how to establish power places on your own. You naturally don't have to just depend on yourself to do so. That is beyond human possibilities. But the guardians of many existing, larger power places and other subtle friends are glad to help you carry out such plans if your intentions are pure and all beings with whom you are involved will experience something good in the sense of the cosmic laws. How do you do this?

First, while following the ritual described above, go to a power place with which you have worked for a longer period of time. Explain your wish to establish a new power place when you are there. Describe the place that you have selected for this purpose. Ask if it is suitable. If not, ask for guidance in finding a better one. Then ask for something to create the linking of the new power place to be built with the one that already exists. Take these messages with you and bring them to the place chosen to be the new power place as soon as possible. Using the technique described above, make contact with your Inner Child, your Higher Self, and the Higher Self responsible for the area selected. Explain your intentions to these three and ask for their support. Then make contact with the Higher Self of the power place from which you have brought the message. Now bury the object at the place or put it there in a way that is lasting and concealed from unknowing access there. Request the blessing of the creative force for this plan by lifting your left hand to the heavens and placing the right hand on the ground of the power place. Then also ask Mother Earth for her blessing by bringing the palms of both hands into contact with the ground. Then, place one hand—it doesn't matter which one—on your heart, stretch out the other arm with the palm of the hand turned away from you. Say out loud while you slowly turn around your own axis clockwise one time:

*I ask for the assistance, the protection, and the guidance of the powers of light and love, the beings of nature and the elements. Everyone is welcome here who seeks healing and knowledge, protection and help, loving care and power to better serve the good of the Creation or who would like to give support to these intentions.*

Leave one hand on your heart and place the palm of the other hand on your forehead, on your third eye. Feel what is happening within yourself and around yourself for a moment. Now stretch out the arm whose hand was placed on your heart. While doing this, turn the palms of the hands outwards, away from your body. Continue to keep the other hand on your forehead. Now turn slowly around counterclockwise and say out loud while doing this:

*May the blessing of the life forces be here for all eternity, may this place be in the light of love and bring blessing to those whose are dedicated to the power of good. May this place be closed on the subtle levels for everyone and everything that does not support, recognize, and protect the universal order. So be it with the approval of the heavens and the Earth for now and for always, for everything and for everyone.*

Now place both hands on your forehead, close your eyes, and feel what happens. If you like, simply remain for a while at this new power place, surrender yourself to the gradual increase of the vibration in its surroundings, and rejoice with the subtle powers and beings of nature at this new light center. When you go, be sure to stick to the power-place ritual described above. When you return to visit this place again, remember that it is now a fully valid power place and act accordingly.

During the next six months, and naturally longer if you like, make contact with the Higher Self of the new power place time and again and provide it with Reiki energy. This is very important, particularly in the development phase. It's especially good to create such a power place with a group of like-minded people and work together with it.

# Why New Power Places
# Should Be Established

New power places can be established at the meeting places of spiritual groups, in seminar centers, and, if you like, naturally also in your yard or in a park if you live in a city. However, they can also have beneficial effects in other places.

Today there are so many regions in our world that urgently could use more contact with the subtle powers and their healing possibilities. These may be power plants or waste dumps, the places in which political or economic decisions of great scope are made, or those in which drug dealers do their dirty business and dangerous drugs are consumed, limiting people in their freedom and destroying their health. The problems of our world are often so complicated that there perhaps are no direct, conventional solutions for them.

*Our most important problems cannot be solved on the same level in which we have created them.*                    (Albert Einstein)

Structures must be changed, values transformed, and the abilities of consciousness, personal responsibility, and the ability to love must be continually developed. With Rainbow Reiki you can help. Establish new power places at the focal points of difficulties or close to them and look after them. Activate and strengthen the existing places of power. Work together with the Higher Selves, the subtle beings, and the powers of light, love, nature, and the elements for global transformation. They need us human beings in order to become extensively and lastingly active on this level of existence. We need them because we cannot solve the problems that we have created or cannot solve them satisfactorily enough on our own. This work with the life forces should not take the place of the customary environmental protection and other efforts to let the world and everything on it become more intact. My dream is a holistic concept that includes anything that could help.

Do you want to dream with me? Do you want to have these dreams come true? The tools and the know-how are waiting for you. Use them with much fairness, integrity, and as well as you can. Many hands are necessary. Much must be done in order to once again give the creative force a place on Earth. Let's get started. Now!

# CHAPTER SIX

# Reiki Essences
# A New Method for Discovering the Healing Powers of Nature for Yourself

This chapter is probably the most important one for you in this book. It deals with a (r)evolutionary new method of Second Degree Reiki: how to make substances effective exclusively on the energetic level that can, in a diversity of ways, help anyone who takes them or rubs them in. I call these substances that work on the subtle level Reiki Essences. Their effectiveness is not just because of Reiki alone, but also the healing patterns of etheric forces that are suited for extensively regulating, harmonizing, and permitting vital processes to develop. Even just making these remedies is a bit of healing for the person who does this.

## The History of Reiki Essences

After my initiation into the Second Degree, I experimented a great deal with the extensive tool kit of this level of training, as I have previously mentioned. New approaches for working with this method soon developed from my research on Reiki mental healing. One of these was the direct clearing of selected areas of the mental level[34] in minerals, liquids, and other substances. One initial practi-

---

[34] Within the context of the Second Reiki Degree, the mental level is the area of the human mind that automatically, and for the most part unconsciously, processes our sensory impressions (hearing, seeing, feeling, smelling, and tasting) and initiates reactions of a mental, emotional, energetic, or physical type according to given patterns. The programs existing on the mental level are very useful if they take the requirements of our everyday life into consideration. As a result, the conscious portion of the human being obtains the space to deal with new experiences. They become a hindrance, sometimes even dangerous, when reactions that were important a long time ago, such as during childhood, continue to be produced in adulthood and thereby limit a person's competence to that of an earlier age in a certain situations in life. Compulsive revolting against authority, thoughtless subjection, many fears and addictions are examples of older programs that are no longer suited to the current situation in life. Compare this with my comments in *Reiki— Way of the Heart*, Lotus Light.

cal result was the Reiki amulet with stones cleared by special Reiki methods, exercising a harmonizing and healing effect on the person who wears it. However, it wasn't possible to awaken the more extensive, deeper powers in the materials with these methods alone. Because of this, I kept on searching and found the solution for introducing differentiated energetic healing powers into material carriers, through which they can be effective on this plane, in old Vedic and Egyptian writings.

# The Theoretic Background
# of Reiki Essences

Everything that exists on this level is basically a more or less filtered emanation of patterns originating in other dimensions of the Creation. God contains everything that is. The vibrations that communicate with each other to some degree in various forms for certain lengths of time, but never for eternity, come from Him. On the levels of separation, to which our plane of existence also belongs, there are many relationships between the individual parts of the Creation, the effects of which can either contribute to or prevent its development. If there are strong obstacles to development, then a being's structures that carry the vital forces on its level of existence suffer as a result. In order to once again regenerate these, it is meaningful to go one or more levels higher in the direction of the source of all life and bring a type of replacement part from there to the level of the damaged structure. The problem in doing so is moving the replacement part in an undamaged and functional state from one level to the other and bringing it into the damaged structure in such a way that the lasting "repair" is guaranteed. A wonderfully simple and certain way of doing this in many cases appears to be the tool kits of the Second Reiki Degree. With it, protected bridges can be built through which healing patterns can be transported without damage and in full effectiveness to practically every level of the Creation. To do this, nothing material must be destroyed as in many flower essences and homeopathy in order to release these subtle forces.

I differentiate between three levels in the methods explained in this chapter:

1. *The material level*, on which we all live and where we are happy or sad, healthy or sick, and—usually—more or less unconscious in relation to the origin and purpose of our incarnation.

2. *The level of the Higher Selves.* Every part of the Creation on this level of existence has a "Higher Self" assigned to it. People and

some animals such as dolphins, horses, pigs, and apes have an individual Higher Self. Other animals like ants, bees, spiders, as well as plants and minerals, have Higher Selves that are respectively responsible for larger groups or the entire race. A Higher Self contains the life plan of a being. Stored within it are the themes with which it would like to have experiences in its existence here. The respective being has decided on these themes before its present incarnation. No specific destiny is stored within the life plan. There are no stipulations as to who has which experiences with whom and whether happiness or suffering, profit or less is the result. The point of death isn't contained here and neither is a specific goal in life. The same also applies here: the path is the goal. However, special individual strengths and weaknesses are stored here. The degree to which a person develops and lives out his strengths or cures and protects weaknesses is always decided by that individual. This is the gift of freedom that God puts in the cradle of every one of His children.

The original, intact, and individual building plan for every being is found on the level of the Higher Selves. Many patterns for Reiki Essences are tapped here so that they can provide the necessary complicated vibrational patterns on the material level for the re-creation of harmony. Structures for mastering more extensive life crises related to the developmental process can't always be obtained here. When something is required that is truly new for the affected individual, these forces are then acquired from further levels closer to the source of life.

3. This is *the level of the spiritual teachers*, a type of Higher Self of the Higher Selves. The power animals of the shamans can be found here, for example, as well as the beings we call angels or gods—but please don't confuse these with the One God, the source of life.

There are further levels of the Creation suitable for making certain Reiki Essences or with which it is possible to work in this respect. However, a longer, more extensive, and practical involvement with the second and third level are an absolute precondition for meaningful contacts with them.

# Who Can Make Reiki Essences?

Anyone who has been initiated into the First and Second Degree by a Reiki Master/Teacher trained in the spiritual line of Usui-Hayashi-Takata-Furumoto / Dr. Webber-Ray and in the fundamental techniques of energy intensification, mental healing, and distance treatment can make Reiki Essences. If you are in doubt about your training, talk to your Reiki Master and have him explain his line of training and initiation to you. Here is how to make the actual essences:

First, it's important to prepare yourself so that an optimal transmission of healing powers occurs through you.

# Preparing to Make the Reiki Essences with Reiki and Meditation

The long preparation for making Reiki Essences through Reiki and meditation exercises explained in this section will probably try your patience a bit. But in your own interest, please make them exactly like they are described here. The channels for the enormous subtle forces required for making the Reiki Essences have high demands. When you have made the Reiki Essences on a regular basis for some time, meaning at least one to two per week for three to four months, such extensive measures beforehand will no longer be necessary. You will feel it. In case of doubt, play it safe and adequately prepare yourself. No objective harm can occur to you if you go into the making of an essence without preparation. However, it is possible that the essence won't work or that you experience strong healing reactions. The reason for this can be energetic blocks that sit very firmly. When they are suddenly dissolved, strong fluctuations of feelings, increased sensitivity, or trance states can also temporarily occur in case the energetic power of your hara is inadequate for emotionally stabilizing you as intensively transmit clarifying vibrations.

When I write a book like this, I must put a great deal of trust in the reader, which means you, responsibly dealing with the information published here. What you do with it is up to you. I can only show you the way and give you the best map possible as orientation for the journey—but you have to walk it alone. If you don't take to heart the map and the directions for the way, the road can become quite bumpy.

The following steps represent the fundamental preparation for making Reiki Essences. During this time, please do without coffee, black tea, alcohol, and at least reduce your nicotine consumption if you smoke. In terms of your diet, skip pork and reduce the portion of meat that you eat. Even better would be to eat a vegetarian diet for this week. Take a walk for at least 30 minutes a day and drink 2 liters of water. These measures help channel the blocks, waste products, and metabolic poisons out of you and thereby intensify the effect of the meditation and Reiki treatment.

***Step 1:***

a. For one week, give yourself a whole-body treatment with Reiki or let a friend give you Reiki every day.

b. During this week, carry out an *additional* hara meditation[35] for at least fifteen minutes every day by sitting with a straight back and properly positioned pelvis on a chair. Your head should be held as if a thread was attached to the top of it and gently pulled towards the sky. Now breathe into your lower belly, about two fingers beneath your navel. This is the approximate location of your hara, a type of vital-energy reservoir and balancing organ of a subtle nature. Breathe calmly, deeply, and evenly. Imagine that streams of energy are flowing into your hara every time you inhale, that they collect there, and that every time you exhale the depleted energies that hinder the flow of the life force within you stream out of you and once again return to the eternal cycle of vital energies. At the end of every meditation, give yourself about one minute of Reiki on the lower belly. More doesn't hurt.

c. Give your Higher Self and your Inner Child about 15 minutes of Reiki every day by way of distance contact. You can treat both of them separately or also at the same time for this purpose. Even if you have completed the fundamental preparation for making the Reiki Essences described here, you should send the two of them at least 15 minutes of distance Reiki once a week in order to maintain and constantly expand the willingness to make this remedy.

***Step 2:***

In the following week, give yourself a chakra energy balance with Reiki every morning and evening by placing one hand on the 1st chakra and the other on the 6th for about five minutes. Then do the same with the 2nd and 5th, followed by the 3rd and 4th energy center.

After this phase of preparation, if your are not seriously physically or psychologically ill, you should be capable of dealing with making the Reiki Essences. But please be sure not to take on too much for yourself! First make one essence and then wait two or three days to see what effect it has on you. If you do well with it, try using two every day. You should only make more than three es-

---

[35]In my training sessions on the Reiki essence method, I use the three-ray meditation, which can be worked with in a much more effective manner in this context, instead of this. Unfortunately, you can only learn this through initiation, which I why I describe the hara meditation here. Transcendental meditation or kriya also functions quite well for this purpose.

sences a day when you have had a great deal of practical experience with them and your reactions to them.

Directly before making an essence, give yourself a whole-body treatment with Reiki and carry out the hara meditation for 15 minutes. After making one or more essences, repeat the 15-minute hara meditation and give yourself a chakra balance with Reiki. If you regularly make essences more than twice a week, a chakra balance before and about five minutes of the hara meditation afterwards are enough.

If you don't make any Reiki Essences for a longer period of time, but you would like to be ready to do so without any extensive measures and have completed the basic preparation described above, give yourself a whole-body treatment with Reiki every week and carry out the hara meditation for about 15 minutes once along with it (see Step 1).

## Making Reiki Essences in General

You will need a suitable carrier substance for the following technique. I most often use white refined sugar. Brown sugar will do, but it usually doesn't accept as well as white sugar. Instead of sugar, you can also use water. Water from the tap is okay if it is filtered. Don't use distilled water! If you want to store the liquid essence for a longer period of time, don't forget to preserve it with alcohol. You can get 90% alcohol for this purpose in any pharmacy. If you have worked with Bach Flower Essences, you will be familiar with this. If you want to play it safe, boil the water and the container for the Reiki essence in advance. The essences—whether solid or liquid—can be kept in the dropper bottles available at pharmacies in various sizes. If you want to make a Reiki Essence ointment, sweet almond oil or jojoba oil are well-suited for this purpose. Pharmacies and alternative cosmetic stores have these products and the proper containers to keep them in.

Keep in mind that you shouldn't make portions that are too small. The same amount of time, about 30 minutes, and Reiki needed to create 25 ml of Reiki Essence is also enough to make 250 ml. For more than a half liter, double the amount of time. This will then be enough for up to 2 liters of essence. However, you will seldom need this much since the Reiki Essences are used sparingly.

About five hours before you make a Reiki Essence, don't drink any alcohol or the like. For about one hour before, don't eat any chocolate or drink chocolate milk. Stop smoking and don't drink any more black tea or coffee. Wait at least one hour after you have made the essence before you consume alcohol or the like and at least 30 minutes before you smoke, drink coffee or black tea. Before the preparation, you should wash your hands with soap and water up to about the middle of your lower arm.

### Step 1: Charging the giver pattern

Using the distance-treatment symbol and the energy-intensification symbol, as well as the corresponding mantas, initiation a Reiki distance treatment. Direct the flow of energy by calling the recipient's name three times. Hold the palms of your hands turned away from you, and don't visualize anything in particular regarding the recipient, which is normally a Higher Self. If you see something in front of your inner eye, that's fine. If not, that's okay as well. Request cooperation. Explain your intentions of making a lastingly effective Reiki Essence on a certain theme (which you should describe as briefly and precisely as possible) to the giver of the healing pattern. Then request to have its healing pattern made available to you. In exchange, offer it Reiki and intensify the flow of Reiki several times through the corresponding symbol and its mantra. Continue to request support, loving care, and protection when making the Reiki Essence. Then give the recipient Reiki for at least 15 minutes. The power on the other end of the line will often inform you on its own when the charging is adequate. Thank it.

### Step 2: Channeling healing powers

Now attach a mental-healing symbol and an energy-intensification symbol over the carrier substance. Use the corresponding mantras to activate the signs and then say the name of the carrier substance either out loud or in your mind three times. For example: "This water, this water, this water." The type of container that the carrier substance is in or its material isn't important for the success of energy transmission. However, to store it for a longer period of time, you should use one made of glass.

Now request the force that you have called to send the healing vibrational pattern. Wait until the energy has flowed completely through you into the carrier substance. You will feel that it is finished by a subsiding of the flowing or another clear sign. However, the process should generally be completed after a maximum of 20 minutes. If you should be interrupted while you are making the essence and have to remove your hands and do something else, again start at the beginning of establishing contact and charging.

Now the new Reiki Essence is finished and ready to be used.

# Reiki Essence Dosage

*To take it orally*, please dilute the Reiki Essence made according to the process described above in a relationship of 1:20 for people who react very slowly and of 1:100 or more for people who easily react to subtle healing forces. One to five drops daily, distributed throughout the day, can be taken over a longer period of time to achieve the desired results. In case of doubt, it's better to use a lower dosage and stronger dilution. People who have never taken a Reiki Essence should have just one drop in a glass of water and drink it distributed the period of one day. Then wait for about 14 days and carefully observe the reactions. It's quite possible that this dose is totally adequate for the respective person. If nothing has happened, check to see whether the essence was the correct one since if the quality given to the person isn't the proper one, it naturally won't do anything. If it's the right one, slowly increase the dose and pay attention to the reactions.

*To rub it in*, dilute the charged Reiki Essence to a relationship of at least 1:50. As needed, use one or more times daily. If the person has never used a Reiki Essence, only rub it in once and wait 14 days for the reactions.

You can also compare the issue of dosage with the report of the experiences by the healing practitioner and Reiki Master, Anne Witt in the Appendix Two.

**Please observe:** For about three hours directly after the first administration of a Reiki Essence, the person given the treatment shouldn't do any activity that requires powers of concentration and a normal state of consciousness. An example of this would be driving a motor vehicle or operating heavy machinery. It has sometimes been observed that a type of healing trance occurs within this stated period of time. This isn't a drug trip, but is based on the sudden release of strong subtle energies and the healing restructuring in the body, mind, and energy system that they cause. When we know how the affected person reacts to the respective Reiki Essence, would can tailor it more individually. However, in case of doubt, play it safe.

# Examples of Preparation and Effect of Various Reiki Essences

## 1. Making Transformation Essences and their effects

Transformation Essences are usually created through the contact with the Higher Self of an individual, usually the maker of the essence.

**Process:**[36]

**Step 1:** Establish contact using the distance-treatment symbol and the energy-intensification symbol, as well as the corresponding mantras.

**Step 2:** Clearly direct the flow of energy by stating the name of the recipient—Higher Self of (your first and last name, Higher Self of (your first and last name, Higher Self of (your first and last name)—three times. Keep the palms of your hands turned away from you with the intention of finding your subtle partner there somewhere and don't visualize anything in particular about the recipient.

**Step 3:** Respectfully request it to support your intentions of making a lasting Reiki Essence with an effect, such as "joy in living", and offer Reiki in return for it.

**Step 4:** Send distance Reiki to the Higher Self for about 15 minutes to give it the power to bring the healing pattern to this plane through you.

**Step 5:** Attach a mental-treatment symbol and an energy-intensification symbol over the carrier substance, sugar, for example, and use the corresponding mantras in order to active the signs.

**Step 6:** Clearly direct the mental healing by stating the name of the carrier substance three times—for example: this sugar, this sugar, this sugar, and looking at it.

**Step 7:** Ask your subtle partner to now put the healing energy pattern into the carrier substance through you.

**Step 8:** Wait until the stream of energy has flowed through you completely. According to my experience, this practically always happens after about 20 minutes.

**Step 9:** Thank the giver of the healing pattern, ask it to work with you again the next time, and correctly end the distance contact. *In no case should you maintain it during the entire period of time required for the complete creation of a Reiki Essence!*

---

[36]Also compare with "Making Reiki Essences in General," further above.

# Examples of Proven Transformation Essences

As an impulse for you, now I'll give a more detailed explanation of some of the Transformation Essences and list a series of other interesting essences of this type without explaining their details. You can also compare these with the Pendulum Tables in the Appendix.

## Energy Balance

This essence dissolves imbalanced collections of vital energy that aren't chronic within a relatively short time and thereby promotes the balanced, natural flow of the vital forces, making it easier to work with the deeper blocks and disharmonies. Useful for shock, life crises of all types, fear, emotional imbalance, travel sickness, headache, and digestive disturbances, as well as intensive healing reactions. This is similar to the Rescue Remedy of the Bach Flowers in many respects.

## Basic Trust

Some people are lacking in the fundamental trust in life. This essence can help to promote the deep trust that is necessary to be happy, deal with all types of problems in a more relaxed manner, and not let oneself be thrown out of an inner attitude of security in the turbulence of everyday life.

## Joy in Living

This essence supports the ability to be joyful, to play, and happily enjoy yourself like a child. In contrast to most other essences that I know of, it works quite quickly and effectively for many people. After you have taken it, don't drive a car or do anything requiring a great degree of seriousness for three to four hours. When you have gathered more experience with this remedy, you will know how to best deal with it on your own.

## Flexibility

This essence can help people who have a very rigid way of living their lives, don't look to the left or to the right, are possibly intolerant, and can't learn anything because they cling too much to what is familiar to them.

## Letting Go

Some people make their lives more difficult by not being able to let go of what has become unnecessary in order to make room for something new. This essence is also helpful for stinginess, fear of being devoted or letting oneself go as a precondition for relationships, or for the free flow of feelings in relationships.

## Accepting

Appropriate for the helper syndrome, poverty consciousness, and the inability to learn. Sometimes beneficial for so-called "therapy-resistant" people; however, you should check the qualifications of the therapist extensively beforehand. Perhaps the problem is to be found here.

## Divine Order

Use this when everything within a person is chaotic, he simply can't find his place in the world and the friends and relationships appropriate for him. Useful for everything that blocks or twists the natural order in the body, mind, and soul. However, this isn't a universal remedy since a concrete formation of new relationship structures with oneself and others, as well as the mastering of the related, completely normal problems in life, must always follow. *Divine Order* is a type of basic essence for the successful treatment of many problems, a first step in the right direction.

## Ability to Love

The ability to love means being able to resonate with other people and things in a cheerful, trusting, and interested way. This doesn't mean wanting to be there for everything and everyone and sacrificing oneself. The commandment of "love your neighbor *as yourself*" also has something to do with this. If a person can't accept himself and many other people and things in a warmhearted way, is hateful, greedy, envious, jealous, fearful, arrogant, intolerant, cruel, or full of feelings of competition, this Reiki Essence will help.

## Meaning of Life

The *meaning of life* can't be found in a rational way. It can only be felt and sensed. The ability to do this is like the keel of a sailboat: it stabilizes the voyage and makes it possible to cross against the wind. This essence helps in giving one's own life a direction and a task.

This doesn't concern objectives, but rather a person's right path on which he comes into contact with the demands and successes, phases of relaxation, and insights that fit him alone and no one else in the suitable manner and at the right time.

## Grounding

This essence can help harmonize headaches, dizziness, an excess of subtle impressions, as well as a lack of interest in the demands and completely normal things of everyday life like friends, a partner relationship, sex, money, profession, property, health, one's own physical nature, and the like.

## Heavening

This is the right remedy if a person doesn't want to deal with anything that creates comprehensive insights into his life and the course of the world; if he is only interested in power, money, possessions, sex, the tangible world, and everyday life; and if he is lacking in creativity, activity, curiosity, and flexibility.

## Awaking

Some people move through the world as if they were in a deep hypnotic trance. They have no idea what's going on, have a ponderous way of thinking, act as insensitive as an elephant in a china store, have accidents because they are daydreaming, and the like. This is also appropriate for addictions, drug abuse, and problems that are constantly talked around—and thought about—and for co-dependency. Supportive for every type of consciousness-developing and clarifying psychotherapy. But not a substitute for it!

## Further Examples

Endurance, Assertiveness, Willingness to Develop, Decisiveness, Relaxation, Peace, Patience, Willingness to Act, Willingness to Heal, Humor, Intuition, Ability to Concentrate, Creativity, Willingness to Learn, Courage, Openness, Responsiveness (frequently a suitable successive remedy for Ability to Love: promotes the development of subtle perception and the ability to live in harmonious relationships), Feeling of Self-Worth, Tolerance, Responsibility, Forgiveness.

## II. How to Make Plant Essences

Wonderful Reiki Essences can be made from all types of plants. At the same time, their effect isn't necessarily identical with that of the Bach Essences or similar essences, phytotherapeutic agents, or remedies produced in a homeopathic manner. However, the effective components of all preparations are contained in the respective Reiki Essences. They are complemented by further qualities that are in part not yet known and only become available through this special way of making the essences. Also compare this with the respective Pendulum Tables in Appendix Four. No material components are necessary here either. However, it is beneficial to have seen and touched the corresponding plant at least once.

### Making the Essences

Do **Step 1** as explained under I. Also do **Step 2** as explained under I., but direct the energy flow by calling the "Higher Self of (add name of the plants—for example: the birch)" three times. Do **Step 3** as under I., but with the intention of creating a lastingly non-perishable Reiki Essence with the effect of (add the name of the plant). Do **Steps 4 to 9** as explained under I.

There is still much to discover in the area of plant essences. Because of the abundantly available literature on this topic, I refer you to the Commented Bibliography in the Appendix, with the restrictions mentioned above. In the books there you will find more detailed explanations of the healing powers of many plants than I can give because of the limited space.

## III. Making Healing-Stone Essences

Reiki Essences with a versatile spectrum of effects can be made from every stone and every mineral. In the process, the effect isn't necessarily identical with the healing-stone essences made in the customary manner, but they contain many of their components. A discussion of how the various remedies work would take us too far afield at this point. Please look at the related Pendulum Tables in the Appendix Four. You should also have seen and touched the respective healing stone at least once here as well.

### Making the Essences

Do **Step 1** as explained under I. Also do **Step 2** as explained under I., but direct the energy flow by calling the "Higher Self of (add name of the type of stone or mineral, for example: the rose quartz)" three times. Do **Step 3** as under I., but with the intention of creating a lastingly non-perishable Reiki Essence with the effect of (add the name of the stone or mineral). Do **Steps 4 to 9** as explained under I. It is beneficial to have been in the physical proximity of the respective healing stone at least once.

## IV. Making the Power-Animal Essences

Every type of animal has a Higher Self that is responsible for it, even if it belongs to a species with individual Higher Selves. According to my experience, the Higher Self of a species represents a so-called power animal or medicine animal. For many native peoples and those who work shamanically, the healing powers, the special knowledge, and the many other important abilities of these subtle beings have been valued for millennia. Subtle beings are very friendly and willing to help human beings if they are treated with respect and sincerity. It is said that every person has at least one power animal as a companion and if he accepts it and requests help in mastering the crises in his life, it will support him to the best of its abilities. Power animals are neither all-powerful nor all-knowing, yet they can be good friends, advisors, and teachers to us human beings in many respects.

Power-animal essences are excellent remedies for working through extensive problems for which you don't know where you should start in solving them. You must choose the appropriate power animal before making such an essence. It is normally not helpful to rationally determine the giver of such Reiki Essences unless you have extensive shamanic knowledge and experience. The oracle principle has proved itself to be much more suitable for this purpose. Get yourself about 30 to 50 cardboard cards of the same size. Write down the name of a different animal and draw a picture of it—or cut it out somewhere and paste it—on each of the cards. If you would like ready-made cards, the *Medicine Cards* by J. Sams and D. Carson from Bear & Company are well-suited for this purpose. Along with the set of cards, there is also a book giving precise descriptions of the qualities of each of the power animals. Another possibility is using the pendulum to determine the appropriate power animal. You will find the corresponding Pendulum Tables in Appendix Four.

### *Selection of a Power Animal*
### *for an Essence According to the Oracle Principle*
Take 15 minutes and be sure that you won't be disturbed. You might want to light an incense stick and do the hara meditation for several minutes in order to separate yourself from the everyday world and become attuned to the spiritual work that will follow.

Ask the question: "Which power animal can help me solve the problem (add a description of the problem)?" Think of the question while you shuffle the cards, lay them out in a concealed position, and draw one of them. Now you know which power animal thinks it can contribute to clearing up your difficulties. Thank it for having made itself known to you and request its help.

### Making the Essences
Do **Step 1** as explained under I. Also do **Step 2** as explained under I., but direct the energy flow by calling the "Higher Self of (add name of the animal species, for example: the deer )" three times. Do **Step 3** as under I., but with the intention of creating a lastingly non-perishable Reiki Essence with the effect of (add the name of the animal species). Do **Steps 4 to 9** as explained under I.

## V. Making the Angel Essences
Angels are subtle beings that are actively concerned with tasks related the development and maintenance of the Creation in general, as well as that of individuals. We are most familiar with the four archangels: Gabriel, Michael, Raphael, and Uriel, but there are a great number of others. A useful introduction to the world of angels is offered by the set (book and cards) called *Angel Blessings* by Kimberley Marooney, Merrill-West Publishing, Carmel, CA., 1995.

Please note: The archangel essences, as well as those of some of the other angels, often have a very dynamic effect. At the beginning, apply them with at least twice the normal level of dilution you use for other essences, put one drop of the dilution in a glass of water, and only let the person drink a small swallow of it. Observe the reactions for at least three weeks before you think about giving the essence again.

### Selecting an Angel for An Essence
Take 15 minutes and be sure that you won't be disturbed. You might want to light an incense stick and do the hara meditation for several minutes in order to separate yourself from the everyday world and become attuned to the spiritual work that will follow.

Ask the question: "Which angel can help me solve the problem (add a description of the problem)?" Think of the question while you shuffle the cards, lay them out in a concealed position, and draw one of them. Now you know which angel thinks it can contribute to clearing up your difficulties. Thank it for having made itself known to you and request its help. Also compare the respective Pendulum Tables in the Appendix Four for selecting an angel.

### Making the Essences

Do **Step 1** as explained under I. Also do **Step 2** as explained under I., but direct the energy flow by calling the angel (add name of the angel, for example: Archangel Gabriel) three times. Do **Step 3** as under I., but with the intention of creating a lastingly non-perishable Reiki Essence with the special power of the angel or with the energy quality that it finds most suitable for the healing of your imbalances. Do **Steps 4 to 9** as explained under I.

## VI. Making the Organ Essences

For every organ, it's possible to make a Reiki Organ Essence that can give normalizing impulses to the corresponding part of the body. Also see the corresponding Pendulum Tables in the Appendix Four.

### Making the Essences

Do **Step 1** and **Step 2** as explained under I. Exception for Step 2: Should the essence not be effective or not have a satisfactory effect, direct the distance contact to the Higher Self of the person who would like to take the organ essence. Do **Step 3** as under I., but with the intention of creating a lastingly non-perishable Reiki Essence with the effect of normalizing the specified organ, such as the liver. Do **Steps 4 to 9** as explained under I. A very interesting and versatile organ essence is:

### Thymus

This is suited as a remedy for revitalization in order to prevent premature symptoms of aging, strengthen the immune system, indirectly stabilize the heart function, and for general strengthening.

## VII. Making General Chakra Essences

I understand general chakra essences to be Reiki Essences that have a normalizing and developing effect on one of the major or minor chakras. When selecting a chakra essence, consult the Chakra Pendulum Table in the Appendix Four.

### Making the Essences

Do **Steps 1 and 2** as explained under I. Do **Step 3** as under I., but with the request for help in creating a lastingly non-perishable Reiki Essence with a healing and developing effect in particular for a chakra (add the name of the chakra, for example, the 2nd chakra). Do **Steps 4 to 9** as explained under I.

## VIII. Making Planetary and Stellar Reiki Essences

Under these essences I understand the healing pattern of the Higher Selves of the planets, such as Venus, Mars, or Jupiter, the Higher Self of the Moon or specific astrological constellations, such as Aquarius, and naturally also our Sun or our home world, the Earth.

Please consult the books mentioned in the Commented Bibliography of the Appendix for the effects of these types of Reiki Essences. There are some very good ones on this topic that can better and more extensively explain the various energy qualities of the planets and constellations than it is possible for me to do here.

### Selecting a Planetary or Stellar Higher Self

If you would like to attempt to make an astrological card set for selecting a heavenly giver suited for working on a respective problem, this is naturally quite useful for reasons similar to those applying to the Power Animal and Angel. When doing so, please observe the rules that I have explained in detail under the points above. There are also corresponding Pendulum Tables in the Appendix. If you know a good astrologer, he can also give you competent tips for selecting the astrological vibrational pattern for you at a certain point in time or in general.

### Making the Essences

Do **Step 1** as explained under I. Also do **Step 2** as explained under I., but direct the energy flow by calling the "Higher Self of (add name of the planet, astrological constellation, Moon, etc., for example: Venus)" three times. Do **Step 3** as under I., but with the intention of creating a lastingly non-perishable Reiki Essence with the effect of (add the name of the planet, astrological constellation, the Moon, etc.) or with an energy quality that it finds useful for solving your problem. Do **Steps 4 to 9** as explained under I.

## IX. Making Metallic Reiki Essences

Metals have been used as a material in homeopathic potencies, as well as in energetically effective elixirs, for many years by experienced specialists. Through the Reiki Essence method, not only the familiar, but also significantly more extensive possibilities for applying the healing subtle vibrations of metals arise.

### Making the Essences

Do **Step 1** as explained under I, as well as **Step 2**, but direct the energy flow by calling "Higher Self of (add name of the metal) three times. Do **Step 3** as under I., but with the intention of creating a lastingly non-perishable Reiki Essence with the effect of (add the name of the metal). Do **Steps 4 to 9** as explained under I.

### X. Examples for Other Types of Reiki Essences

While observing the rules for making Reiki Essences explained above and illustrated in the points I. to X. with many examples, you can craft such remedies from almost every model with which you have at one time come into contact on the material level—if the giver isn't a subtle being. It's worth experimenting with this. Some suggestions are:

Oxygen, Christ, Buddha, runes, Tarot cards, I Ching hexagrams, power places like the Cheops Pyramid, spiritual teachers who are important to you like Jesus, Yogananda, Babaji, or Sathya Sai Baba.

# How Can Reiki Essences Be Used Everywhere and What Should Be Observed in the Process?

Not only human beings can resort to the help of Reiki Essences in minor or major health problems or other problems in life—they are also very good for plants and animals. Try it out!

Please remember that you bear a great deal of responsibility for the use of this knowledge. Respect other people's freedom to decide and never give them something of the essences without their express permission. This wouldn't be right and certainly not spiritual. If you can't ask because the respective being isn't capable of speech, plants, animals, small children, and people in comas, for example, establish contact with the responsible Higher Self and ask whether you are permitted to work with a Reiki Essence in relation to this being. Feel what's going on inside yourself and respect the answer! Take this comment on your personal responsibility very seriously in your own interest!

# An Application of the Reiki Essence Method for Advanced Students

In closing, here is a further interesting area of use for the Reiki Essence method. However, you should only use it if you have gathered abundant experience in making Reiki Essences and knowledge about their effects.

Just as you can channel the energy of a giver's Higher Self into a carrier substance, it's naturally also possible to directly use this to treat a person or some other being. To do this, charge the giver's Higher Self for just 30 seconds to a maximum of 2 minutes and explain to it that it should formulate the harmonizing vibrations to directly treat a person or other being and not for making a Reiki Essence.

In order to achieve a holistic effect, it's appropriate to transmit the power to the respective person through the position used for mental healing with Reiki, specifically the initiated hand on the top of the head and the other on the medulla oblongata at the center of the back of the head.

The healing power can naturally also flow to every other area of the body by a direct laying on of the hands or within the scope of a distance treatment. However, it will then only have an effect in the respective area. But this can also be quite useful for certain reasons. For example, to release the rest of the energy system from a largely isolated trauma, such as phantom limb pain.

*Please pay attention to the following chapter* before you begin your practical work with the essences. It contains a great deal of things worth knowing about healing reactions, professional training possibilities, and what should be observed in legal terms when it comes to giving the essences to others.

# CHAPTER SEVEN

# Reiki Essences
# in Practical Application

There are a number of useful or even necessary things you should keep in mind when using the Reiki Essences. You will find information about them in this chapter.

## What Happens
## When Reiki Essences Are Used?

When a person becomes healthy in a natural way or even if he effectively works on himself in a spiritual sense, healing reactions will occur. If it is clear that this will happen and is taken into consideration, there should hardly be any greater problems as a result. However, someone who isn't properly prepared for this may become fearful or falsely appraise what is happening and not react appropriately.

Furthermore, it may be that one Reiki essence for treating an imbalance is not sufficient or that it hasn't been suitably selected and therefore shows no results. It's important to not exceed one's own level of competence here, be sure to consult an experienced medical professional *in time*. This topic will be discussed in detail below.

## What Are Healing Reactions?

A healing reaction is the body's response to something normalizing its vital energies. The following may occur in individual cases:

a. A detoxification process takes place on the physical, emotional, mental, and energetic level. As long as toxins and waste materials of all types are not removed from the body, it can't truly become healthy. As long as old, bottled-up feelings aren't expressed, they inhibit the flow of other current feelings. As long as a person lives his life in a way that doesn't lastingly fulfill his individual needs and doesn't make growth possible for him, or constantly weakens him, it won't be possible to maintain his health and well-being. When energies that have long become inappropriate are stuck in his chakras or meridians, he won't be able to properly develop himself in the spiritual sense or in other ways.

All the points mentioned here are naturally connected with each other.

Nothing can be dissolved in isolation without at least starting to bring other things into the living flow.

b. Suppressed and chronic afflictions of all types become acute for a time and their symptoms manifest themselves more intensively. In the larger sense, this process is also part of detoxification.

c. Restructuring takes place on all levels. This can temporarily create a feeling of insecurity, loss of the sense of being safe and secure, difficulties in making decisions, emotional fluctuations, diminished mental and emotional powers of endurance and initiative, as well as greater emotional vulnerability. Once the new structure has been created, a considerably higher degree of endurance, stability, creativity, and joy in living arise.

d. The processes mentioned under a. to c. require a great deal of energy and suitable material for building the new physical structures. This means that more sleep, less stress, an increased intake of liquids to support the metabolism and detoxification, light and regular exercise, and easily digestible, healthy food with considerably more vital substances are required than normally.

# Social Impact of Taking Reiki Essences

The observation has frequently been made that taking Reiki Essences supports not only the development of the individual who takes them, but that there are subsequently effects on other people who are frequently together with him and inwardly prepared for opportunities of growth. People are connected with each other and with other beings in their daily environment in many ways and not just on the subtle and energetic level. In this respect, it's understandable that far-reaching development processes of a person in a relationship can positively influence the other partner if he or she isn't closed to meaningful changes.

So please don't be surprised if things get moving in the right direction for the partner, other members of the family, colleagues, or close friends. But don't count on this happening every time!

# When Should You See a Doctor?

As a non-professional, you can use the Reiki Essences within the scope of home and family health care for yourself and your loved ones, as well as in a preventive manner, for experiencing your self and developing your personality. *For all cases of serious illness—no matter what type—and for everything where you are uncertain whether it could be serious, you must absolutely consult an experienced medical profession* in order to have a correct diagnosis made and, if necessary, an appropriate therapy prescribed and its effects monitored. Traditional Reiki, the advanced methods of Rainbow Reiki and other approaches can possibly be used as accompanying therapies. Inform the doctor providing treatment if you would like to take additional action and coordinate this with him.

If there are initial changes for the worse and these don't disappear within three days or are very severe, a medical professional should also be consulted to be on the safe side. It may be possible to weaken a vehement healing reaction through simple measures or there might be another illness that needs to be treated concealed behind the presumed healing crisis.

# Interaction of Reiki Essences with Other Medications

To the best of my knowledge, there are no direct interactions of Reiki Essences with chemical or natural medications.

In homeopathic treatments, it is often no longer possible to clearly define the additional effect of a Reiki essence in relation to that of the homeopathic remedy. It isn't clearly apparent which of them had the actual effect. For this reason, a patient should consult the medical professional giving him homeopathic treatment before taking a Reiki essence.

The effects of some medicines may be reduced through the detoxifying action of Reiki Essences. This is only dangerous when the medications must be maintained at certain levels within the body in order to insure survival. If such medications are taken or it isn't clear whether they are necessary for survival, the doctors providing the treatment must unconditionally be consulted before taking the Reiki Essences. Discuss what should be taken into consideration with respect to the prescribed medication when the body has improved its ability to detoxify itself.

If organs function better as a result of using the Reiki Essences, it may be necessary to reduce or terminate use of the medication supporting one of these organs. Only the doctor providing the treatment can make this decision! For diabetics who must take insulin, life-threatening circumstances may otherwise arise when improved functioning of the pancreas occurs. In all of the cases mentioned, definitely request the advice of the medical professional providing the treatment and have him do follow-up examinations on a regular basis.

## Reiki Essences and Regulations

Every country has its own regulations regarding healing activities in the narrower and broader sense.

Only trained and authorized medical professionals like doctors, naturopaths, and the assisting medical professions like physiotherapists are normally permitted to make diagnoses or prescribe therapies. Any other unauthorized person is liable to prosecution. In my opinion, in addition to the legal perspective, it isn't spiritually and ethically correct for people who are not medical professionals to try to give treatment in the same way as a doctor would.

"Cobbler, stick to your last!" is an old saying that applies here. Otherwise, you should complete a recognized form of medical training and pass an examination bestowing on you the official permission to give medical treatment to people who are seriously ill, if this is what you want to do. Or use your knowledge only with people who are basically healthy.

## One Reservation on My Part...

With publication of the knowledge about Rainbow Reiki in general and the Reiki Essence method in particular, I would like to contribute to the possibility of every person who has the corresponding prerequisites—First or Second Degree Reiki—of working privately for himself and his family with it and receiving a benefit from it.

I don't want any type of economic activities, production, application, seminars on the topic, written information, videos, sound carriers, and the like to be developed under the terms Reiki Essence, Rainbow Reiki, or Rainbow Reiki Mandala by people who haven't been instructed by me personally or by teachers who I have commissioned to do so. They should be instructed in the theory and practice of Rainbow Reiki and authorized to do this work. This is the only way I can have some guarantee that nothing else is passed on to unsuspecting people under these terms. For this reason, I have had the terms mentioned here legally protected in Germany and other countries.

# Certification Training
# at the Reiki-Do Institute

For medical professionals, the Reiki-Do Institute Walter Lübeck offers certified training in making and using Reiki Essences and other Rainbow Reiki methods suited for the medical practice in cooperation with experienced medical professionals.

# Training for Non-Professionals
# in the Reiki Essence Method

Non-professionals can also receive training in the Reiki Essence method for their own private needs. The Reiki-Do Institute Walter Lübeck offers seminars and workshops on this topic, as well as diverse teaching material.

# A Brief Introduction of the Four Aura Fields and Seven Major Chakras

## A Survey of the Human Subtle Energy System

### The Aura Fields

*The Etheric Body:* Information about the physical structure; access to the universal life energy; ability to feel and act in the subtle area.

*The Emotional Body:* Carrier and organizer of the emotional life and the instincts. Stores emotional energies that aren't expressed.

*The Mental Body:* Carrier and organizer of the conscious and unconscious thought processes, as well as the mental habits such as valuations, ethical and moral ideas.

*The Spiritual Body:* Connection of the human being with the creative force, the point of unity for all life.

### *The Major Chakras*

*1st Energy Center*—Root Chakra: survival, preservation of the species, structure, struggle. Organs: bones, nails, teeth, adrenal glands, legs, blood.

*2nd Energy Center*—Sexual Chakra: joy in life, closeness, ability to be in a relationship, desire and physical expression. Organs: urogenital system, kidneys, skin, arms, fluids in the body.

*3rd Energy Center* —Solar Plexus Chakra: power, dominance, fear, karma, separation, analytic thinking. Organs: digestive system, liver, solar plexus, autonomic system, joints, tensed state of the musculature, energy metabolism, detoxification processes through elimination/encapsulation.

*4th Energy Center*—Heart Chakra: love, unity. Organs: heart, parts of the pancreas, thymus gland, detoxification through storage in fatty deposits, relaxed state of the muscles.

*5th Energy Center*—Throat Chakra: self-expression, individuality, communication. Organs: throat, nape of neck, lungs, thyroid gland, balance between physical and mental-emotional-spiritual growth.

*6th Energy Center*—Forehead Chakra: perception of one's individual path within the cosmic context. Organs: ears, nose, eyes, pituitary gland.

*7th Energy Center*—Crown Chakra: cosmic consciousness, transformation, ecstasy. Organ: pineal gland.

### The Minor Chakras

*The Yin Chakra:* Similar to, but much less flexible and complicated in function than the 7th energy center, the crown chakra. Connection to unity with everything that is yin on both the inside and the outside

*The Yang Chakra:* Similar to, but much less flexible and complicated in function than the 7th energy center, the crown chakra. Connection to unity with everything that is yang on both the inside and the outside.

*The Nutrition/Responsibility Chakras:* These energy centers regulate every type of responsibility, as well as nutrition in the material, energetic, and informative area.

*Hand Chakras:* Expression of the energies of all chakras in the outer world and perception in the subtle area.

*Elbow Chakras:* Regulation of the intensity of relationships. For example: being able to accept people and things and draw boundaries.

*The Knee Chakras:* Ability to teach and learn. Devotion to life with all the consequences or to death.

*Foot Chakras:* Function similar to that of the hand chakras, but instead of being directed at other living beings, the connection to the Earth stands in the foreground here. Harmonious, grounded development of spirituality and material happiness.

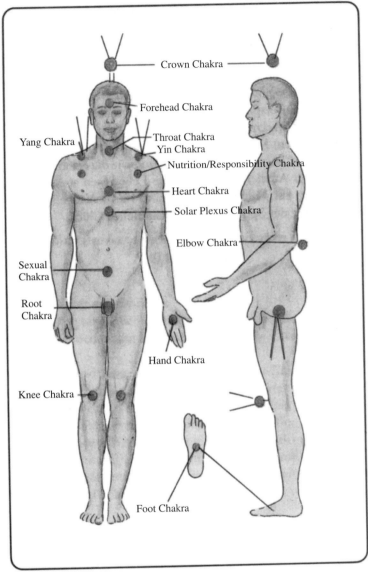

*Major and minor chakras*

137

# Experiences with Reiki Essences

## By Anne Witt, Healing Practitioner and Reiki Master

### *Notes on the decoder dermatography interpretation*

Lead 7 shows the condition of the 1st chakra, lead 2 that of the 2nd chakra, lead 4 that of the 3rd chakra, lead 6 that of the 4th chakra, lead 1 that of the 5th chakra, lead 3 that of the 6th chakra, and lead 5 that of the 7th chakra. The red "flags" represent the first measurement (initial value without reaction stimulation), the green the second measurement after the reaction stimulation by the measuring devise, and the blue represent the values after administrating the Reiki essence (therapeutic intervention). In the optimal case, the green flag should extend beyond the red flag. The green flag reflects the regulatory ability of the organism after stimulation by the measuring device. If the stimulation is taken well by the body, it is "healthy." The less the body can regulate this, the more imbalanced it is at this time.

### *Case 1: A patient who has experienced sexual abuse*

She was given the essence "Release of the Abuse Theme." Dosage: 1 x daily 3 drops. Several days after taking the drops, a discharge of pus from the paranasal sinuses and coughing with pain in the heart area occurred. The patient also continued to take the drops during these reactions. She interpreted it to be cleansing and excretory reactions. Changes began to take place in her partner relationship. It became clear that the partner also had problems with the abuse theme. Communication on this topic was initially difficult, and the partner decided to also go into psychotherapeutic treatment in order to deal with his share of the problem. During this time, I provided psychotherapeutic care for the patient and supported the process with chakra work using the metamorphic method. The physical symptoms subsided after some time without having to use any further medications. In a biophysical examination, it was determined that the problem of the karmic partner relationship began to be resolved. We are still awaiting the further results.

Evaluation: I made the Reiki Essence for the various energy bodies. This process has very clearly shown a deep-reaching and quick, in part also dramatic change, of her difficult theme. It was naturally also necessary to provide care for the patient outside the normal practice hours as well. The current healing process became very clear to her, and she showed great willingness to integrate the changes into her life.

Six weeks after the start of treatment with Reiki Essences: the partner relationship has drastically changed. The partner has come into a very strong contact with his inner self for the first time so that the relationship can become deeper. (Note by Walter Lübeck: It is clear here that the effect is not just limited to the person receiving treatment, but can manifest itself as an impact and response in his/her outer world.

### Case 2: A patient with changes in the cells of the cervix
On the basis of a decoder dermatography transcription, a shift in the acid-alkali balance is shown in favor of the acid. In addition to a classic homeopathic remedy, she received the Reiki Essence "Regulation of the Acid-Alkali Equilibrium" for the mental and spiritual, emotional, etheric, and physical level. It should be mentioned here

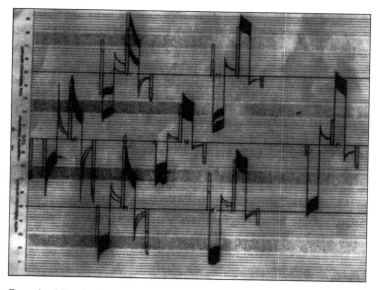

*Example of decoder dermatography printout*

that acid is classified with the masculine principle and alkali is classified with the feminine principle.

The patient reported that she was able to be much less aggressive in dealing with her fellow human beings and her partner. She was able to understand aggression from the outside and no longer needed to emotionally experience this compulsively as being directed against her. She also developed more sympathy for the people she encountered in an aggressive manner, but this type of interaction has occurred less frequently. I advised the patient to regularly treat her uterus with Reiki II, which the patient likes to do on a regular basis. Whether the cell changes have been normalized has not yet been established since the treatment was not complete when this report was written.

### Case 3: A patient with sexual problems
She received the Essence "Solution of the Sexual Problems." One day after taking it, swelling and itching of the labia occurred, which continued for about one week. The second night, four men appeared in her dreams who were apparently involved in the development of her sexuality. The patient was able to let these things arise with a good feeling and is naturally being given psychotherapeutic care.

### Case 4: A handicapped young man
He received the Reiki Essence "Grounding." Three weeks after he started taking it, his mother stated that he could now participate in and tolerate his physiotherapeutic treatments for twice as long. The process is certain to continue.

After a few weeks, the patient came to my practice for scar-clearing. He permitted me to touch him and was quite calm and relaxed about it. At any earlier point in time, this wouldn't have been possible since he had had intense fears of closeness.

### Case 5: A young woman with intensive heart palpitations, a slight alcohol problem, and depressive moods in which she quickly reacted with fear
The patient received the Reiki Essence "Calmness." One week after she started taking it, she reported that the heart palpitations had greatly subsided. In addition, her problems that she had with her parents became more conscious. Now she is calmer when facing them and has achieved more distance to them. She drinks alcohol much less frequently. The patient has been given additional support with energy work and spent a long time in psychotherapeutic group therapy.

*Case 6: A patient involved a great upheaval in life*
*and the resulting confusion and lack of clarity*
The patient received the Reiki Essence "Light and Clarity." At the next therapy session one week later, she reported that many things related to her situation had become clear to her. She sees the direction in which her development appears to be going and has more courage to make decisions. My observation is that she frequently speaks of "clarity" during our conversation.

*Case 7: A patient has problems with her children*
She can't devote herself enough to them, has difficulty tolerating their neediness. The patient received the Reiki Essence "Healing of the Heart Chakra." I carried out a decoder dermatography recording with the patient. The picture shows blocks in leads 2, 4, 5 (intensively over-energized because of an acute cold) and 7, partial blocks in 6 with signs of scarring (could be physical or psychological scars in the heart). After administration of the Reiki Essence, the blocks dissolved according to the decoder recording in lead 2, in part in 4, 6, and 7. While attuning myself to the patient, I had the intuition that the heart chakra should be treated. Then the partially blocked 2nd chakra, which is also responsible for certain areas of the ability to have relationships, could normalize itself as well. The decoder picture confirmed this. Three weeks after the woman had taken the Reiki Essences, her daughter became ill with measles. Something appears to have "tipped the balance" in the situation. Some days later, the patient herself became ill with a feverish infection. She hadn't had a fever for a longer period of time. This was accompanied by coughing, swelling of the lymph nodes in the groin area, and intense toothache without any physical findings, meaning it had an energetic origin. It was noticeable that the patient came into my practice with her daughter and the daughter snuggled up to her mother the whole time without this apparently disturbing her. Her manner of speaking and her appearance also seemed to be softer. The further course must also be awaited here since the healing process has not yet been completed as I write this.

*Case 8: A patient with strong tensions*
*in the entire skeletal musculature*
The tensions has taken on such dimensions that there have been changes in the skeleton, causing intense states of pain. This is conspicuous in the psychological picture since there are relationship difficulties in the broader sense. The patient is very receptive to other people's problems, yet communicating about her own themes is difficult for her. She received the Reiki Essence "Healing of the

142

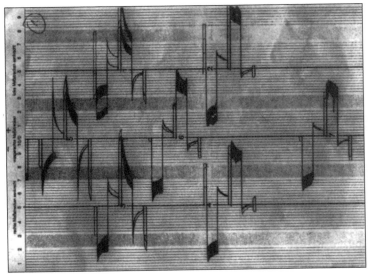

*Decoder dermatography printout for case 7*

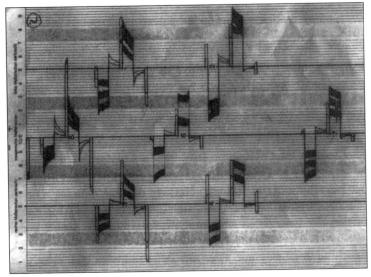

*Decoder dermatography printout for case 8*

143

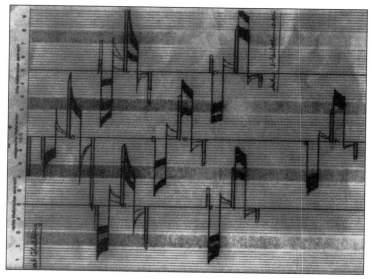

*Decoder dermatography printout for case 9*

2nd Chakra." Under stimulation, the initial decoder picture (red and green) shows a strong regulation in lead 6 (heart chakra), a drop of the energy in lead 2 (2nd chakra: the signs of scars, which could be physical as well as psychological). In lead 7, a drop in energy occurred under stimulation and administration of the Reiki Essence (we must wait for the reaction). The measurement directly after administration of the Reiki Essence shows that the energy of lead 2 (2nd chakra) was already regulated somewhat higher, the energy in the lead 4 (solar plexus chakra) and lead 6 (heart chakra) drops. I associate this with the fact that the patient participated too strongly in other people's suffering and thereby became too far removed from herself. In the next session after one week, the patient reported on exactly this theme. She was now more sympathetic than commiserating and was better able to express her own needs and concerns, which was reflected in an energy increase in lead 1 (5th chakra). The patient felt quite well taking the Essence, and her strong tensions were clearly reduced. Now she can move in way that had been impossible for her for a long time.

### Case 9: A patient with severe abdominal pain during menstruation

The patient has problems in feeling and setting limits and constructively applying her energy for herself and others. The decoder picture shows a block in lead 2 (2nd chakra). I didn't evaluate the over-energized picture in leads 1, 3, and 5 here since the patient had a bad cold. She received the Reiki Essence "Healing of the 2nd Chakra." The direct subsequent measurement showed that the block in lead 2 opened, the energy in lead 4 (solar plexus), 3, and 1 was increased. At the consultation 4 weeks later, the patient reported that she is beginning to set boundaries, which is very clearly expressed in the way her mother had injured her daughter's boundaries. She is more capable of going into the outside world with her energy (energy increase in lead 4) and can more quickly talk about and express this (energy increase in lead 1). She can better open herself for suggestions on thinking about the correlations of her complaints and achieves more insight (energy increase in lead 3); she understands that this theme is a large field of learning for her and that she can develop boundaries not against something, but for herself.

### Case 10: A patient with relationship problems

He strongly withdraws when facing personal confrontations with his partner. I made 2 decoder pictures: the first was created before he took the essence, and the second 2 months later. The first picture shows a clear energy drop in the leads 2, 4, 6, and 7; lead 3 (6th chakra) shows a block, reflecting his lack of insight for his share of the theme. When measured again after 2 months, a clear energy change was shown. An increase of energy had taken place in all of the leads that had previously been weak, the block in lead 3 had been dissolved (the patient shows clearly more understanding of his share). He has been able to develop more sympathy and understanding for his partner. We will keep an eye on the leads 2 and 3 and their psychological theme since it is desirable for these to become more strongly regulated.

### Case 11: A patient who has had amalgam removed

The patient received the Reiki Essence "Detoxification." The initial decoder measurement shows an energy drop in the leads 4, 6, and 7. In these leads are the excretory organs on the physical level. After administration of the essence, the energy increased in the leads 4 and 6, and increased somewhat in lead 2. The weakening in lead 7 presumably represents the patient's ovulation that has just occurred; the over-energized leads 1, 3, and 5 reflect the currently existing parasinal infection, which had previously existed as a chronically latent process.

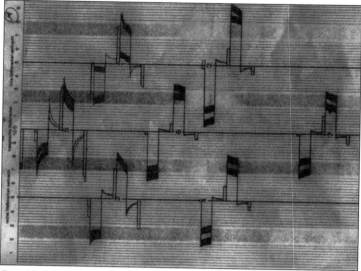

*Decoder dermatography printout for case 10a*

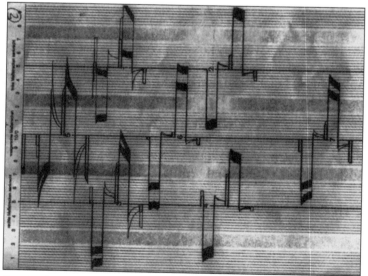

*Decoder dermatography printout for case 10b*

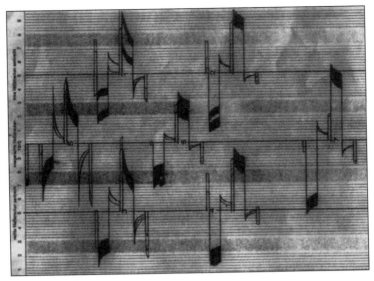

*Decoder dermatography printout for case 11*

# General Observations
# on the Reiki Essences in My Practice

The Reiki Essences appear to work on a very deep level and are apparently capable of resolving karmic themes. The transformation takes place at a tempo that is hardly imaginable. It's very much like a quick-motion effect. In my opinion, this is why it's necessary for those who use the Reiki Essences to deal with them and the people who take them in a very responsible manner. I think that an experienced naturopath/psychotherapist should watch over the healing process when there is a serious physical and/or emotional and mental illness or when it looks like there is a greater imbalance. Qualified training in making, selecting, and applying the Reiki Essences should be an obvious preparation for anyone who wants to deal with them professionally. It's necessary to understand and competently accompany the healing and growth processes triggered by the Reiki Essences in order to bring them to a "round" conclusion. People who aren't familiar with the natural course of holistic healing processes or are only superficially aware of them could otherwise wrongly evaluate the reactions to the treatment of severe imbalances with Reiki Essences, reacting with fears that could hinder the progress of the healing. Emotional healing crises require accompaniment, if only just to keep the consciousness of what is happening in step with the actual occurrences and offer a shoulder to lean on. In times of profound developmental processes, every individual needs a social environment that supports and understands him, stabilizing him from the outside during the time of transformation since his inner life is in chaos. A new, more healthy order is then created during the course of the healing.

# Reiki, Shamanism, and Working with the Healing Powers of Nature

### By Greta-Bahya Hessel-Lübeck, Reiki Master and Shaman

Working with the power of nature, with Reiki, and the traditional shamanic methods is a part of my everyday life. I train people in shamanic healing methods and have been permitted to gather a variety of experiences with the combination of different energy systems together with my students.

## What is Shamanism?

Shamanism is one of the oldest and most basic systems of healing. Before there even were doctors, male and female shamans were the healers of the society. For shamans, nothing is without a soul. By respecting the other parts of the world and deeply loving them, they can heal relationships and help dissolve separations. Shamanism spread out from India to Siberia into the whole world, only to be suppressed in the so-called advanced civilizations through institutionalized religion.

Unfortunately, people today have largely lost access to these archaic powers. Through our technology and performance-oriented society, the soul suffers increasingly from stress and estrangement from itself, other people, and nature. Allergies, cancer, AIDS, and artificially triggered environmental catastrophes threaten humanity and cause fear and pain. In view of these threats, human beings are searching for ways out of the suffering. Shamanism offers many paths for this purpose, and so it has once again become relevant. Old rituals are now coming to life because people need them, and the modern world painfully misses them.

# What Shamanism Isn't

Unfortunately, there are also a great many communication problems on the topic of "shamanism." Some people consider shamanism as a possibility for dropping out and withdrawing from society because they can't deal with it or have worked themselves into an "end-of-the-world" mood. On the other hand, there are other people who think it's the official permission to take drugs. Many people simply try to live out their power through what they call "shamanism." Others in turn have totally left the solid ground of reality and find themselves in a constant state of delirium, confusing "tripping out" with shamanism. However, shamanism isn't an ego trip, but has the objective of a meaningful life together for all beings of the world. Individual characteristics are not only tolerated by it, but desired since they make the happiness of each individual possible and enrich the community with their many unique talents.

# My Path with the Powers

After many years of examination and research, I have developed my own spiritual path. As a philosopher, I quickly understood at the university that perception without experience has no value and that experience without perception makes just as little sense. So I connected the perception (philosophy) with the experience (shamanism). The same results from masculine and feminine ways of thinking: reason—intuition. For the past two-thousand years, societies in most parts of the world have been determined by patriarchy. The patriarchy has set the tone in these times and defined the social structures. The consequence of this is that we are now destroying ourselves and nature. Now we are approaching a new age which, I believe, will be oriented towards androgyny. Feminine and masculine portions can now be integrated meaningfully on the personal and societal levels. The connection of masculine reason and feminine intuition is the shaman within us; it is the reconnection or connection to nature. In our current society, the masculine portion in human beings is primarily lived out. This includes: craving for success, possession, striving for artificial progress without consideration of its effects on the totality of life, analyzing, ruling, and having power. In contrast, feminine values are: intuition, creativity, beauty, relationships, joy, feelings, letting go, sensing, perceiving, softness, being in the flow of life and letting yourself be carried by it. I now see my tasks as bringing people to their feminine aspects through experience and perception so that they are animated within their bodies and happy with themselves, in relationships, and within their environment.

When I met my husband Walter, I found myself on the shamanistic path of initiation. I had gone through long, difficult initiation processes and had succeeded in freeing myself from my self-imposed isolation pattern. Through Walter, I became familiar with Reiki and found out that we had both taken a similar path, but by using different techniques in part. I learned to use the Reiki methods in my shamanistic activities. Since Reiki, as a non-polar, loving energy, is available to everyone who opens up to it through initiation and offers techniques of subtle communication in a simple manner, I can make the shamanistic path and the connection to the healing powers of nature accessible to a great many more people, without them necessarily having to go through the long clarifying processes of suffering beforehand. Increasingly more people who had been involved in the 1st, 2nd, and 3rd Degree with Walter came to my seminars since they wanted to continue to work on themselves, find out more about themselves and more extensively learn about the possibilities of using Reiki together with the healing powers of nature. While shamans work with tobacco or mantras, the Reikians give Reiki in exchange for the support of the spirits. A feeling of security like that of a large family, in which every individual could open up and be accepted with understanding, quickly arose in my groups. On the basis of these preconditions, it was possible for me to contribute to the triggering of profound processes of development that helped master life crises and strengthen body and spirit to such a degree that previous imbalances disappeared. The transformation of the participants happened so rapidly that I often couldn't believe it myself. After one or two seminars, many people looked much clearer and were completely changed in appearance. Everyone had mystic experiences, communicated quite normally with the natural forces, which passed perceptions on to us that we would never have achieved in any other way. We had many experiences beyond the realm of everyday life. For example, as we worked with Reiki on our medicine wheel, someone went to the stone of the thunderbird in order to receive help there and it actually thundered in the sky at the same moment.

# The Medicine Cards in Personal Counseling and Shamanistic Work

The direct connection between Reiki and shamanistic work began with *The Medicine Cards*. During the initiation seminars of the First Degree, I did personal counseling for the participants during the breaks for a while. But I usually didn't have much time available, and the people's problems were large and complicated. So I thought of a method for them to work with the power animals without having much knowledge about shamanism. For this purpose, I selected the oracle game *The Medicine Cards* from Bear & Company. I used these during the consultation by asking the person what problem he had at the moment. We talked about it for a while and then worked out an appropriate question together in order to more closely illuminate the circumstances surrounding the problem. Then I had the client draw one of the concealed cards while he thought of the question. The power animal pictured on the chosen card showed the further path for solving the problem. I read the text on this from the accompanying book, used my shamanic ability to experience more about the problem and its background, and then explained the correlations to him. Afterwards, a leading question could be asked: "Which power animal can I call on to help solve my problem?" The power animal on the card subsequently drawn was then responsible for directly working through the difficulty. We once again read the explanatory text together, and I explained the information. Now the practical work with the power animal could begin. The client was to now obtain a picture or figure of the power animal and give it Reiki for ten minutes a day with his hands, requesting help while doing so. In this way, he created a transpersonal connection with the power animal, thereby giving it Reiki in exchange for its help. Every subtle being of nature greatly appreciates this[37]. The participants had astounding success with this method. If you don't believe it, just try it out yourself. I wish you much success and joy with it.

---

[37] Please don't confuse this technique with the distance-treatment method of the Second Degree. With distance treatment, a certain contact can be made with everything and anyone at any time. With the application described above, contact can only be made with one subtle being that is willing to work with you and is already informed about this work, of which there must at least be a symbolic material picture, and which has already had experience with human beings.

# Pendulum Tables

The pendulum tables should help you work with the methods of Rainbow Reiki in a more structured manner. By working with them, you can receive suggestions for making Reiki Essences, fundamental advice for dealing with a personal problem theme (Table 14), and much more.

Please remember that every person can make mistakes in any activity! Using the pendulum is very useful, but you would be falsely advised if you were to blindly trust the information given to you by the pendulum. Personal responsibility is also the key to the successful use of a method here—which applies to dealing with any type of spiritual tools as well.

The information of "Error" is listed in every pendulum table. If the pendulum swings there, use Pendulum Table 2 "Error Correction" in order to get a more detailed picture of the error.

Pendulum Table 1 should help you determine a basic path for solving a difficulty. Then consult the corresponding section of this book in order to obtain further information and work with the other pendulum tables.

In the Commented Bibliography (Appendix Five), you will find a series of books, that will help you learn more about a plant, power animal, or metal, for exemple.

And now I want to wish you much enjoyment and success in using the pendulum!

# Pendulum Table 1

## Basic Rainbow Reiki Work Methods

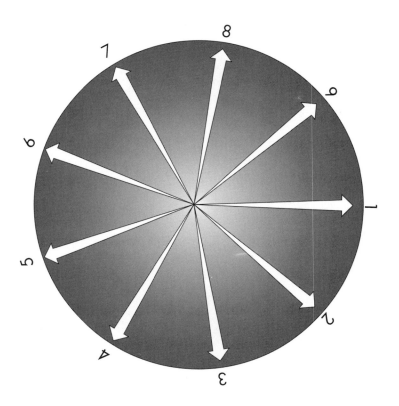

1. Error Correction Table
2. Reiki Essences
3. Rainbow Reiki Plant Mandalas
4. Rainbow Reiki Healing-Stone Mandalas
5. Power-place work
6. Work with the Higher Self
7. Work with the Inner Child
8. Work with power animals
9. Work with other subtle helping forces

# Pendulum Table 2

## Error Correction

1. Outer disruptive influences
2. No trust
3. Prejudice
4. No serious interest
5. Answer not on this table
6. Vanity
7. Incompetent
8. Not concentrated
9. Too tired
10. Disruptive magical influence
11. Respect the privacy of others
12. Answer isn't permitted at this time
13. Error

# Pendulum Table 3

## Reiki Essences

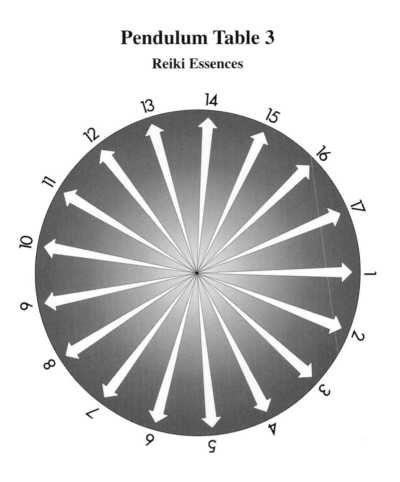

1. Transformation Essence
2. Stellar Essence
3. Power-Animal Essence
4. Healing-Stone Essence
5. Organ Essence
6. Plant Essence
7. Metal Essence
8. Angel Essence
9. Chakra Energy-Card Essence
10. General Chakra Essence
11. Planet Essence
12. Error
13. Element Essence
14. Meridian Essence
15. I-Ching Essence
16. Rune Essence
17. God Essence (Krishna or Tara, for example)

# Pendulum Table 4

## Healing Stones

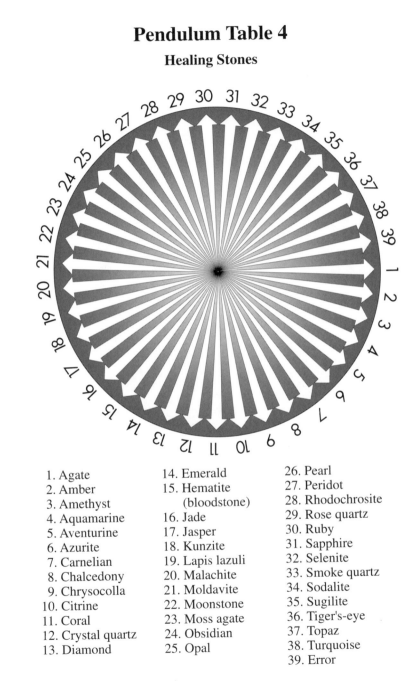

| | | |
|---|---|---|
| 1. Agate | 14. Emerald | 26. Pearl |
| 2. Amber | 15. Hematite | 27. Peridot |
| 3. Amethyst | (bloodstone) | 28. Rhodochrosite |
| 4. Aquamarine | 16. Jade | 29. Rose quartz |
| 5. Aventurine | 17. Jasper | 30. Ruby |
| 6. Azurite | 18. Kunzite | 31. Sapphire |
| 7. Carnelian | 19. Lapis lazuli | 32. Selenite |
| 8. Chalcedony | 20. Malachite | 33. Smoke quartz |
| 9. Chrysocolla | 21. Moldavite | 34. Sodalite |
| 10. Citrine | 22. Moonstone | 35. Sugilite |
| 11. Coral | 23. Moss agate | 36. Tiger's-eye |
| 12. Crystal quartz | 24. Obsidian | 37. Topaz |
| 13. Diamond | 25. Opal | 38. Turquoise |
| | | 39. Error |

# Pendulum Table 5 A

## Power Animals

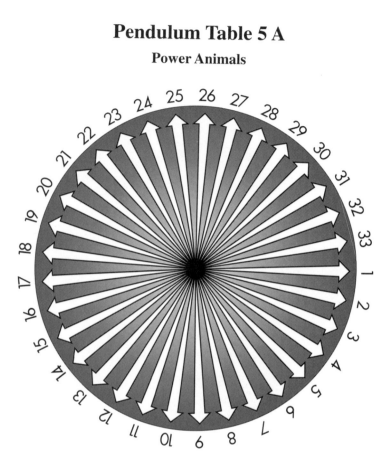

| | | |
|---|---|---|
| 1. Ant | 13. Crane | 25. Frog |
| 2. Antelope | 14. Crow | 26. Goat |
| 3. Ape | 15. Deer | 27. Goose |
| 4. Armadillo | 16. Dog | 28. Power-Animal |
| 5. Badger | 17. Dolphin | Table B |
| 6. Bat | 18. Dragon | 29. Error |
| 7. Bear | 19. Dragonfly | 30. Griffin |
| 8. Beaver | 20. Eagle | 31. Hare |
| 9. Buffalo | 21. Elephant | 32. Horse |
| 10. Butterfly | 22. Elk | 33. Hummingbird |
| 11. Cow | 23. Falcon | |
| 12. Coyote | 24. Fox | |

158

# Pendulum Table 5 B

## Power Animals

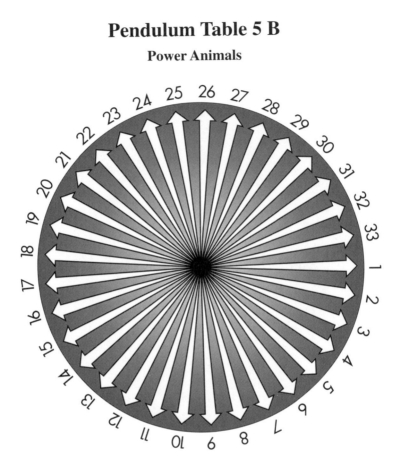

| | | |
|---|---|---|
| 34. Lion | 46. Rabbit | 58. Turtle |
| 35. Lizard | 47. Rat | 59. Unicorn |
| 36. Lynx | 48. Raven | 60. Wapiti |
| 37. Mountain lion | 49. Reindeer | 61. Whale |
| 38. Mouse | 50. Salmon | 62. Weasel |
| 39. Opossum | 51. Seagull | 63. Wolf |
| 40. Otter | 52. Skunk | 64. Woodpecker |
| 41. Owl | 53. Snake | 65. Error |
| 42. Pegasus | 54. Spider | 66. Power-Animal |
| 43. Pig | 55. Squirrel | Table A |
| 44. Porcupine | 56. Swan | |
| 45. Prairie chicken | 57. Turkey | |

# Pendulum Table 6

## Angels

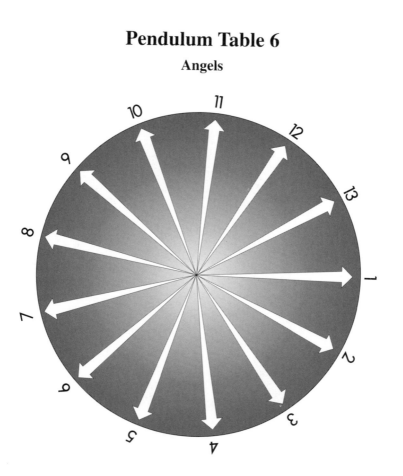

1. Other Angels
2. Error
3. Camael
4. Gabriel
5. Haniel
6. Metatron
7. Michael
8. Raphael
9. Raziel
10. Sandalphon
11. Uriel
12. Zadkiel
13. Zaphikiel

# Pendulum Table 7 A

## Plants

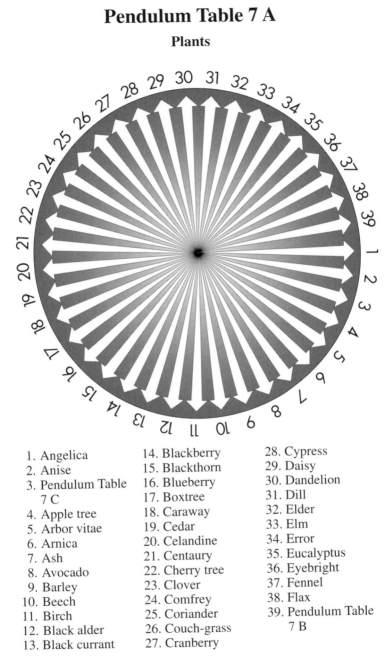

1. Angelica
2. Anise
3. Pendulum Table 7 C
4. Apple tree
5. Arbor vitae
6. Arnica
7. Ash
8. Avocado
9. Barley
10. Beech
11. Birch
12. Black alder
13. Black currant
14. Blackberry
15. Blackthorn
16. Blueberry
17. Boxtree
18. Caraway
19. Cedar
20. Celandine
21. Centaury
22. Cherry tree
23. Clover
24. Comfrey
25. Coriander
26. Couch-grass
27. Cranberry
28. Cypress
29. Daisy
30. Dandelion
31. Dill
32. Elder
33. Elm
34. Error
35. Eucalyptus
36. Eyebright
37. Fennel
38. Flax
39. Pendulum Table 7 B

# Pendulum Table 7 B

## Plants

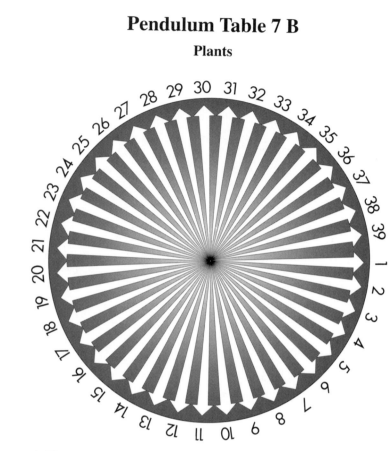

| | | |
|---|---|---|
| 1. Fig tree | 15. Hops | 29. Milk thistle |
| 2. Fumaria | 16. Horse chestnut | 30. Mustard |
| 3. Garlic | 17. Horsetail | 31. Oak |
| 4. Gentian | 18. Juniper | 32. Oat |
| 5. Ginger | 19. Larch | 33. Olive tree |
| 6. Gingko biloba | 20. Licorice | 34. Orange tree |
| 7. Ginseng | 21. Linden tree | 35. Orthosiphon |
| 8. Golden rod | 22. Madder | leaves |
| 9. Hawthorn | 23. Mallow | 36. Pansy |
| 10. Hayseed | 24. Mango | 37. Error |
| 11. Hazelnut tree | 25. Maple | 38. Pendulum Table |
| 12. Herniary | 26. Marigold | 7 A |
| 13. Hibiscus | 27. Marjoram | 39. Pendulum Table |
| 14. Holly | 28. Melissa | 7 C |

# Pendulum Table 7 C

## Plants

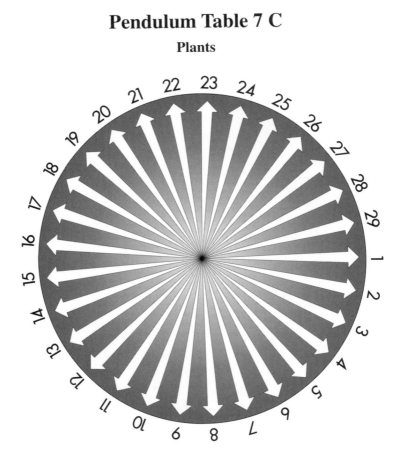

1. Papaya
2. Passionflower
3. Pear tree
4. Peppermint
5. Pine
6. Pineapple
7. Quince
8. Rampion
9. Raspberry
10. Ribwort

11. Rose
12. Rosehip
13. Rosemary
14. Rye
15. Sage
16. Strawberry
17. Tea tree
18. Thyme
19. Wheat
20. White cabbage

21. Willow
22. Wormwood
23. Yarrow
24. Plant not listed
    on the tables
25. Error
26. Plant Table A
27. Plant Table B

# Pendulum Table 8

## Metals

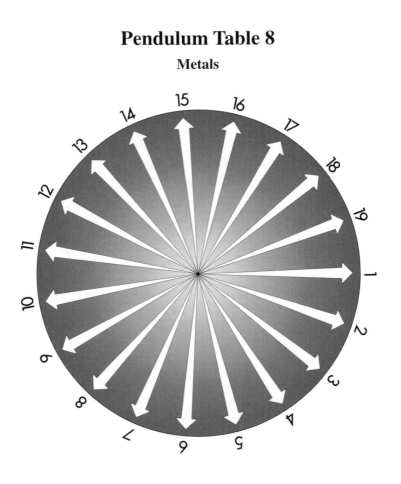

| | |
|---|---|
| 1. Aluminum | 11. Palladium |
| 2. Antimony | 12. Platinum |
| 3. Bismuth | 13. Silver |
| 4. Copper | 14. Tin |
| 5. Gold | 15. Titanium |
| 6. Iron | 16. Tungsten |
| 7. Lead | 17. Zinc |
| 8. Magnesium | 18. Error |
| 9. Mercury | 19. Other metal |
| 10. Nickel | |

# Pendulum Table 9

## Planets and Other Astrological Heavenly Bodies

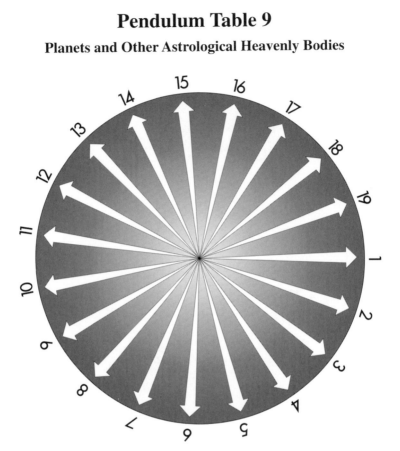

1. Other heavenly bodies
2. Ceres
3. Chiron
4. Earth
5. Error
6. Juno
7. Jupiter
8. Mars
9. Mercury
10. Moon
11. Neptune
12. Pallas
13. Pluto
14. Saturn
15. Uranus
16. Venus
17. Vesta

# Pendulum Table 10

## Constellations

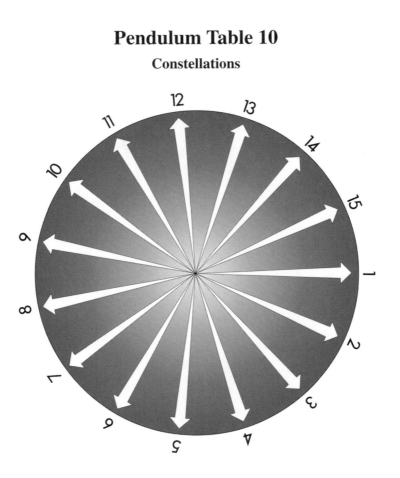

1. Other constellation
2. Error
3. Aquarius
4. Aries
5. Cancer
6. Capricorn
7. Gemini
8. Leo

9. Libra
10. Pisces
11. Pleiades
12. Sagittarius
13. Scorpio
14. Taurus
15. Virgo

# Pendulum Table 11

## Organs

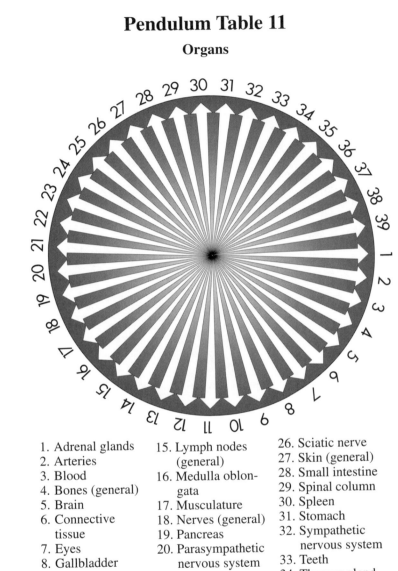

1. Adrenal glands
2. Arteries
3. Blood
4. Bones (general)
5. Brain
6. Connective tissue
7. Eyes
8. Gallbladder
9. Heart
10. Hypothalmus
11. Kidneys
12. Large intestine
13. Liver
14. Lungs
15. Lymph nodes (general)
16. Medulla oblongata
17. Musculature
18. Nerves (general)
19. Pancreas
20. Parasympathetic nervous system
21. Parathyroid gland
22. Pineal gland
23. Pituitary gland
24. Rectum
25. Salivary glands
26. Sciatic nerve
27. Skin (general)
28. Small intestine
29. Spinal column
30. Spleen
31. Stomach
32. Sympathetic nervous system
33. Teeth
34. Thymus gland
35. Thyroid gland
36. Vagus nerve
37. Veins
38. Error
39. Other organ

# Pendulum Table 12

## Transformation Essences

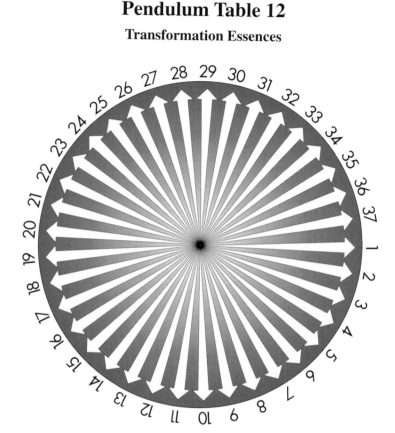

| | | |
|---|---|---|
| 1. Ability to Concentrate | 14. Feeling of Self-Worth | 27. Relaxation |
| 2. Ability to Love | 15. Flexibility | 28. Responsibility |
| 3. Ability to Play | 16. Forgiveness | 29. Responsiveness |
| 4. Accepting | 17. Grounding | 30. Tolerance |
| 5. Assertiveness | 18. Heavening | 31. Vitality |
| 6. Awaking | 19. Humor | 32. Willingness to Learn |
| 7. Basic Trust | 20. Intuition | 33. Willingness to Act |
| 8. Courage | 21. Joy in Living | 34. Willingness to Develop |
| 9. Creativity | 22. Letting Go | 35. Willingness to Heal |
| 10. Decisiveness | 23. Meaning of Life | 36. Error |
| 11. Divine Order | 24. Openness | 37. Other Transformation Essences |
| 12. Endurance | 25. Patience | |
| 13. Energy Balance | 26. Peace | |

# Pendulum Table 13

## Major Chakras

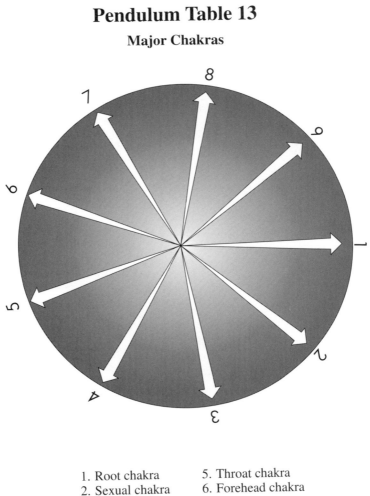

1. Root chakra
2. Sexual chakra
3. Solar plexus chakra
4. Heart chakra
5. Throat chakra
6. Forehead chakra
7. Crown chakra
8. Minor chakra
9. Error

# Pendulum Table 14

## General Advice

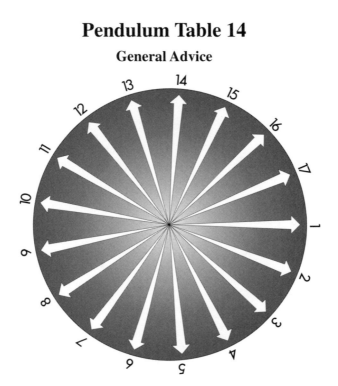

1. More contact with your Higher Self
2. More contact with your Inner Child
3. Use Reiki mental-healing technique
4. Pay less attention to others
5. Pay more attention to others
6. Be nicer to your body
7. Train your consciousness
8. Live out your feelings more
9. Get more exercise
10. Eat a healthier diet
11. Heal your fears
12. Play more
13. Your claims to power stand in your way
14. Learn to forgive
15. Learn tolerance
16. Look for a competent human teacher
17. You lack knowledge
18. You lack experience
19. You need more friends
20. Concentrate on what is important
21. Be more concerned with a fair exchange
22. Error
23. You will find no advice here (at this time)
24. You lack human warmth
25. Your perfectionism stands in your way
26. Satisfy your true needs
27. Look to yourself and not to others

# Commented Bibliography

## Astrology

*Earth Mother Astrology* by Marcia Starck, Llewellyn Publications. Much concrete integration of the astrologic principles. A very good explain on the asteroids used in modern astrology is given as well, along with the zodiac.

*Astrology, Psychology & the Four Elements* by Stephen Arroyo, CRCS Publications. A excellent introduction to modern astrology.

## Aura and Chakras

*Inner Bridges* by Fritz Frederick Smith, Humanics Publishing Group. For advanced readers, a very well-founded book, containing much useful information.

*The Chakra Handbook* by Bodo J. Baginski and Shalila Sharamon, Lotus Light. An excellent book about the functions of the seven main chakras with many exercises, classification tables, and thought-provoking ideas.

## Trees/Flower Essences/Plants

*Flower Essences* by Machaelle Small-Wright, Perelandra, Ltd. Along with interesting descriptions of the production and effects of the various flower essences, the book presents a great deal of information about the subtle spirit of nature and how we should treat it.

## Angels:

*Angel Blessings* by Kimberley Marooney, Merrill-West Publishing, (book and card deck).

## Healing Reactions/Holistic Healing

*A New Model of Health and Disease* by George Vithoulkas, North Atlantic. A wonderful book about disease and health, seen from the holistic point of view. Suitable not only for naturopaths.

## Healing Stones

*The Healing Power of Gemstones* by Harish Johari, Destiny.

## Power Animals

*Medicine Cards* by Jamie Sams and David Carson, Bear & Company (book and card deck). They have been my companions for many years and I don't want to be without them.

*Earth Medicine* by Kenneth Meadows, Element, UK. The author has very good knowledge about shamanism. He knows what he's talking about, and gives us a true spiritual perspective.

## Modern Life Energy Research

*Blueprint of Immortality* by Harold Saxton Burr, Neville Spearman Publishers (The C.W. Daniel Company, Ltd.).

*The Discovery of the Orgone*, vol. I: *The Function of Orgasm* and *The Cancer Biopathy* by Wilhelm Reich, Orgone Institute Press, Inc. Basic literature for life energy research, body therapy, and the practical principles of spirituality. You must read it!

*The Metamorphic Technique, Principles and Practice* by Gaston St. Pierre and Debbie Boater, Element Books, UK. A wonderful introduction to a fantastic self-help method that you absolutely must read. Alone and in combination with Reiki, they will open you up for new worlds.

Other authors: B. Heim, D. Bohm, F. Capra, H. Matayama.

## Natural Agriculture/New Research about Plants

*The Secrets of the Soil* by Tompkins and Bird, HarperCollins, Australia. Some years ago the authors wrote together the best-seller *The Secret Life of Plants*. This new exciting book is perhaps even more important. Through correct behavior it shows us possibilities to help re-balance our planet's ecological system, as well as our own body and spirit. Accompanied by a good bibliography.

## Pendulum

*Dowsing—Techniques and Applications* by Tom Graves, Turnstone Books, UK. Suitable for advanced readers, the book contains many good ideas and much knowledge. Written by an experienced specialist.

*Pendulum Power* by Greg Nielsen and Joseph Polansky.

## Psychology and Psychotherapy

***Body, Self and Soul Sustaining Integration*** by Jack Lee Rosenberg, Humanics Publishing Group. A detailed introduction to modern psychotherapy, also including spirituality.

***Gestalt Therapy—Excitement and Growth in the Human Personality*** by F.S. Perls, The Julian Press. Gestalt Therapy is one of the basic elements of modern psychotherapy. This book gives us a good general idea of this subject.

***Trances People Live*** by Stephen Wolinsky, Bramble Company. Some people keep living in trance, even without drinking alcohol. This book explains how and why this can be ended.

## The Usui-Reiki System

***Empowerment through Reiki*** by Paula Horan, Lotus Light. It describes many of the ideas of holistic medicine in relation to Reiki.

***Dissolving Co-dependency*** by Paula Horan and Brigitte Ziegler, Lotus Light. Reports and experiences show what Reiki can do.

***The Complete Reiki Handbook*** by Walter Lübeck, Lotus Light. A detailed introduction oriented toward the practice of Reiki healing.

***Reiki—Way of the Heart*** by Walter Lübeck, Lotus Light. The book presents the history of modern Reiki and how Reiki may be used as a method for the promotion of spiritual development in all three degrees.

***Reiki for First Aid*** by Walter Lübeck, Lotus Light. Reiki treatment as accompanying therapy for over 40 illnesses with a supplement on nutrition.

***Reiki—Universal Life Energy*** by Shalila Sharamon and Bodo J. Baginski, Life Rhythm. This was the first book about Reiki. It reflects the atmosphere created by Reiki.

## Shamanism/Kahuna

***Urban Shaman*** by Serge King, Fireside Press. NLP, Kahuna, Shamanism, and much more are mixed into an absorbing and informative book.

***Maps to Ecstasy*** by Gabrielle Roth, New World Library. An urban shaman and artist shows us new, old paths of healing.

***Where Eagles Fly*** by Kenneth Meadows, Element, UK. I've already said good things about the author on the previous page. This book shows many *shaman tools* in detail.

*Growing into Light* **by** Max Freedom Long, DeVorss & Company. A classic work about the modern Kahuna method. An absorbing book, containing much useful information.

*Kahuna Healing* by Serge King, Quest Books, USA. Lots of information about Kahuna, written in a modern style with a very practice-oriented approach.

# About the Author

**Walter Lubeck** is a renowned Reiki master, founder and director of the Reiki-Do Institute. He is a bestselling prolific author of classic works on Reiki, as well as books on other healing methods, such as work with Chakra balancing, pendulums, and auras. In the last years he has developed a method he refers to as Rainbow Reiki which includes an unlimited spectrum of applications like channeling, astral travel, making Reiki essences, therapy with precious stones, as well as personality development and wholistic enviromental protection. He has spent many years studying diverse martial arts, meditation, natural healing and energy work of all kinds. Walter Lubeck orients himself in his entire work toward three basic principles: support of personal individual responsibility, development of the ability to love, and conciousness expansion. His goal is to contribute to the betterment of the quality of daily life through spiritual knowledge and thereby to bring man, nature and God in harmony. He lives with his wife, the philospher and shaman Greta Bahya, and child in Weserbergland, Germany in a landscape filled with ancient power spots.

If you would like to contact **Walter Lübeck** and *The Reiki Do Institute*, please write to:

Windpferd Verlag
"Rainbow Reiki"
Friesenrieder Straße 45
87648 Aitrang
Germany

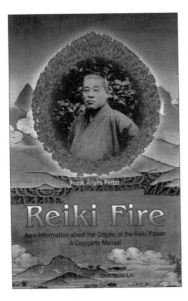

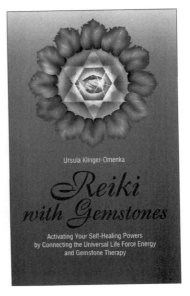

Frank Arjava Petter

**Reiki Fire**

**New Information about
the Origins of the Reiki Power
A Complete Manual**

The origin of Reiki has come to be surrounded by many stories and myths. The author, a free Reiki master practicing in Japan, immerses it in a new light as he traces Usui-san's path back through time with openness and devotion. He meets Usui's descendants and climbs the holy mountain of his enlightenment. Reiki, shaped by Shintoism, is a Buddhist expression of Qigong, whereby Qigong depicts the teaching of life energy in its original sense. An excellent textbook, fresh and rousing in its spiritual perspective and an absolutely practical Reiki guide. The heart, the body, the mind, and the esoteric background, it is all here.

144 pages, $12.95
ISBN 0-914955-50-0

Ursula Klinger-Omenka

**Reiki with Gemstones**

**Activating Your Self-Healing
Powers —Connecting the
Universal Life Force Energy
with Gemstone Therapy**

While Reiki, the universal life energy, brings the physical and emotional functions back into their original harmony, gemstones concentrate light-filled powers and color vibrations into the chakras, whose unrestricted functioning is greatly important for vitality and well-being. By connecting Reiki with gemstone therapy, the powers of self-healing are activated in a natural manner. The author writes on the basis of many years of rich experience in working with Reiki and gemstones. She trustingly places her perceptions into the hands of the reader, who can put them to practical use for the good of all beings within a short time.

128 pages, $12.95
ISBN 0-914955-29-2

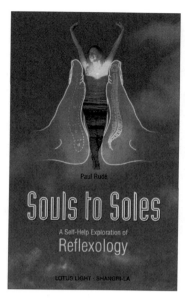

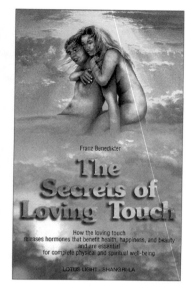

Paul Rudé

**Souls to Soles**

**A Self-Help Exploration
of Reflexology**

Caring for the feet has been part of
the culture of many civilizations, for
thousands of years. Now bursting
forth all over the world, reflexology
is being widely accepted as a safe,
powerful means of reducing stresses,
promoting vitality and well-being.
The author has masterfully captured
the essence of reflexology with beautiful illustrations and clearly presented guides for using your touch
effectively on the feet. Truly an exploration, this book takes you on a
fun loving adventure that has value
for all age groups. Breaking new
ground, this book also shows you
how to reach out to the young, to help
them in their times of discomfort, a
tender loving experience for those
who cannot help themselves.

160 pages, $12.95
ISBN 0-914955-51-9

Franz Benedikter

**The Secrets of Loving Touch**

**How the Loving Touch Releases
Hormones that Benefit Health,
Happiness, and Beauty and Are
Essential for Complete Physical
and Spiritual Well-Being**

Psychologist Franz Benedikter helps
readers create the best possible hor-
monal basis for a healthy, happy, and
liberated life. A release of relaxing,
activating, and euphoretic hormones
occurs when certain trigger zones of
the body are gently touched. With this
compact exercise program, we can
have a positive effect on the body,
mind, and soul through a form of self-
massage and partner massage that
is more like a loving touch. Since
every healthy person has a longing
to be touched, this book introduces
a new age of tenderness.

144 pages, 12.95 $
ISBN 0-941524-90-6

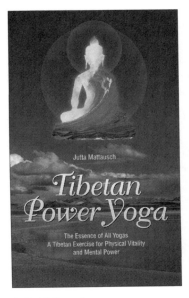

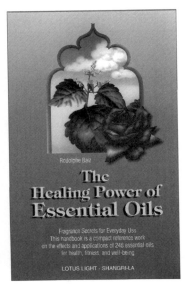

Jutta Mattausch

**Tibetan Power Yoga**

**The Essence of All Yogas
A Tibetan Exercise for
Physical Vitality
and Mental Power**

Here is an absorbing story set in distant Tibet, and yet could also take place within all of us anywhere in the world, since it deals with the journey to the self. Whether you arrive at yourself and then perhaps also find yourself, depends on your willingness to open up ... This completely undogmatic book deals with one of the oldest exercises in the world, an exercise that is simple and unique. "The Tibetan Power Yoga" is what the Tibetan Lama Tsering Norbu calls this set of strong motions, similar to a "great wave" that has given the people from the Roof of the World physical vitality and mental power up into ripe old age since time immemorial.

112 pages, $9.95
ISBN 0-914955-30-6

Rodolphe Balz

**The Healing Power
of Essential Oils**

**Fragrance Secrets for Everyday
Use. This handbook is a compact
reference work on the effects and
applications of 248 essential oils
for health, fitness, and well-being**

Fifteen years of organic cultivation of spice plants and healing herbs in the French Provence have provided Rodolphe Balz with extensive knowledge about essential oils, how they work, and how to use them.
The heart of *The Healing Power of Essential Oils* is an essenial-oil index describing their properties, followed by a comprehensive therapeutic index for putting them to practical use. Further topics of this indispensible aromatherapy handbook are distillation processes, concentrations, chemotypes, quality and quality control, toxicity, self-medication, and the aromatogram.

208 pages, $ 14.95
ISBN 0-941524-89-2

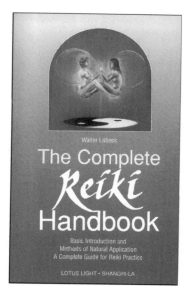

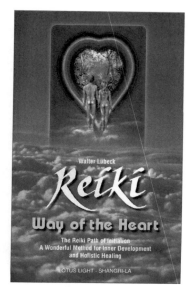

Walter Lübeck

**The Complete Reiki Handbook**

Basic Introduction and Methods of
Natural Application—A Complete
Guide for Reiki Practice

This handbook is a complete guide
for Reiki practice and a wonderful tool
for the necessary adjustment to the
changes inherent in a new age. The
author's style of natural simplicity,
much appreciated by the readers of
his many bestselling books, wonderfully complements this basic method
for accessing universal life energy. He
shares with us, as only a Reiki master can, the personal experience accumulated in his years of practice.
Lovely illustrations of the different
positions make the information as
easily accessible visually as the
author's direct and undogmatic style
of writing. This work also offers a
synthesis of Reiki and many other
popular forms of healing.

192 pages, $ 14.95
ISBN 0-941524-87-6

Walter Lübeck

**Reiki—Way of the Heart**

The Reiki Path of Initiation
A Wonderful Method for Inner
Development and Holistic Healing

*Reiki—Way of the Heart* is for everyone interested in the opportunities
and experiences offered by this very
popular esoteric path of perception,
based on easily learned exercises
conveyed by a Reiki Master to students in three degrees.
If you practice Reiki, the use of universal life energy to heal oneself and
others, you will have the possibility
of receiving direct knowledge about
your personal development, health,
and transformation.
Walter Lübeck also presents a good
survey of various Reiki schools and
shows how Reiki can be applied successfully in many areas of life.

192 pages, $ 14.95
ISBN 0-941524-91-4

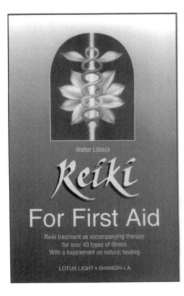

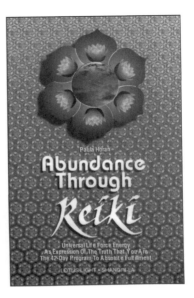

Walter Lübeck

**Reiki For First Aid**

**Reiki Treatment as Accompanying Therapy for over 40 Types of Illness With a Supplement on Natural Healing**

*Reiki For First Aid* offers much practical advice for applying the universal life force in everyday health care. The book includes Reiki treatments for over forty types of illness, supplemented with natural-healing applications and a detailed description of the relationship between Reiki and nutrition.

Reiki Master Walter Lübeck gives extensive instructions on topics ranging from Reiki whole-body treatments to special positions. These special Reiki treatment positions are an important contribution to the field of natural healing.

160 pages, $ 14.95
ISBN 0-914955-26-8

Paula Horan

**Abundance Through Reiki**

**Universal Life Force Energy As Expression of the Truth That You Are The 42-Day Program to Absolute Fulfillment**

*Abundance Through Reiki* is a powerful, poetic evocation of true self and universal life force energy. Its emphasis is a program of 42 steps from Core Self to Core Abundance, creating inner and outer richness. A detailed presentation in the form of two 21-day abundance plans takes you on an exploration of belief patterns that keep you from experiencing everything you need or desire.

Further topics are Reiki and abundance, abundance of health, love, friendship, knowledge, and experience. The book promotes your own natural ability to experience freedom, creativity, and authenticity.

160 pages, $14.94
ISBN 0-914955-25-X

# BIOMAGNETIC
## and Herbal Therapy
## Dr. Michael Tierra

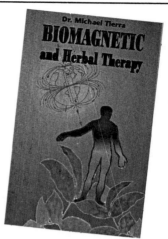

$10.95      96 pp
5 3/8 x 8 1/2 quality trade paper
ISBN 0-914955-33-0

Magnetic energy is the structural force of the universe. In this book the respected herbalist and healer, Dr. Michael Tierra enlightens us on the healing influence of commercially available magnets for many conditions and describes the sometimes miraculous relief from such problems as joint pain, skin diseases, acidity, blood pressure, tumors, kidney, liver and thyroid problems, and more. Magnetizing herbs, teas, water and their usage in conjunction with direct placement of magnets for synergistic effectiveness is presented in a systematic, succinct and practical manner for the benefit of the professional and lay person alike. Replete with diagrams, and appendices, this is a "how to do" practical handbook for augmenting health and obtaining relief from pain.

The paradigm of health in the future is based on energy flow. This paradigm reaches back to the ancient healing arts of the traditional Chinese, the Ayurvedic and the Native American cultures. It is connected to the work of Hippocrates, the "father" of Western medicine, in ancient Greek culture, and found its way through the herbal and homeopathic science that has flourished in Europe over the last few hundred years.

Dr. Tierra is the author of the all-time best selling herbal *The Way of Herbs* as well as the synthesizing work *Planetary Herbology*. He is a practicing herbalist and educator in the field with a background of studies spanning the Chinese and Ayurvedic, the Native American and the European herbal traditions.

To order your copy, ask your local bookseller or send
$10.95 + 3.00 (s/h) to:
Lotus Press
P O Box 325RR
Twin Lakes, Wi 53181 USA

Request our complete book and alternative health products catalogs
of over 7000 items. Wholesale inquiries welcome.

# Sources of Supply:

*The following companies have an extensive selection of useful products and a long track-record of fulfillment. They have natural body care, aromatherapy, flower essences, crystals and tumbled stones, homeopathy, herbal products, vitamins and supplements, videos, books, audio tapes, candles, incense and bulk herbs, teas, massage tools and products and numerous alternative health items across a wide range of categories.*

## WHOLESALE:

*Wholesale suppliers sell to stores and practitioners, not to individual consumers buying for their own personal use. Individual consumers should contact the RETAIL supplier listed below. Wholesale accounts should contact with business name, resale number or practitioner license in order to obtain a wholesale catalog and set up an account.*

### Lotus Light Enterprises, Inc.

P O Box 1008 RR
Silver Lake, WI 53170 USA
414 889 8501 (phone)
414 889 8591 (fax)
800 548 3824 (toll free order line)

---

## RETAIL:

*Retail suppliers provide products by mail order direct to consumers for their personal use. Stores or practitioners should contact the wholesale supplier listed above.*

### Internatural

33719 116th Street RR
Twin Lakes, WI 53181 USA
800 643 4221 (toll free order line)
414 889 8581 office phone
WEB SITE: www.internatural.com

Web site includes an extensive annotated catalog of more than 7000 products that can be ordered "on line" for your convenience 24 hours a day, 7 days a week.